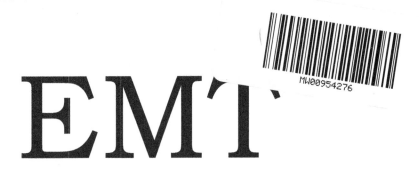
EMT

STUDY GUIDE TEST PREP

2024-2025

Your Toolkit to Achieve Excellence on the First Try! Test | Q&A | Cards | Audio

Elwood Maddox

The following Book is reproduced below to provide information that is as accurate and reliable as possible. Regardless, purchasing this Book can be seen as consent to the fact that both the publisher and the author of this book are in no way experts on the topics discussed within and that any recommendations or suggestions that are made herein are for entertainment purposes only. Professionals should be consulted as needed prior to undertaking any of the action endorsed herein.

This declaration is deemed fair and valid by both the American Bar Association and the Committee of Publishers Association and is legally binding throughout the United States.

Furthermore, the transmission, duplication, or reproduction of any of the following work including specific information will be considered an illegal act irrespective of if it is done electronically or in print. This extends to creating a secondary or tertiary copy of the work or a recorded copy and is only allowed with the express written consent from the Publisher. All additional right reserved.

The information in the following pages is broadly considered a truthful and accurate account of facts and as such, any inattention, use, or misuse of the information in question by the reader will render any resulting actions solely under their purview. There are no scenarios in which the publisher or the original author of this work can be in any fashion deemed liable for any hardship or damages that may befall them after undertaking information described herein.

Additionally, the information in the following pages is intended only for informational purposes and should thus be thought of as universal. As befitting its nature, it is presented without assurance regarding its prolonged validity or interim quality. Trademarks that are mentioned are done without written consent and can in no way be considered an endorsement from the trademark holder.

TABLE OF CONTENTS

INTRODUCTION..9

PREPARATORY...11

EMS Systems...12

Safety and Well-being of the EMT...13
Physical Safety...13
Emotional Well-being..13
Professional Conduct and Ethics..13
Fitness and Health..13
Ongoing Education and Training..13
Crisis and Fatigue Management..14

Medical, Legal, and Ethical Issues..14
Medical Issues..14
Legal Issues..14
Ethical Issues..15

The Human Body..15
The Cardiovascular System...15
The Respiratory System...15
The Nervous System...16
The Musculoskeletal System...16
The Digestive System..16
The Integumentary System..16
The Endocrine System...16

AIRWAY MANAGEMENT...17

Airway Anatomy and Physiology...18
Upper Airway Anatomy..18
Lower Airway Anatomy...19

Basic Airway Management...20
Patient Positioning...20
Manual Airway Techniques and Devices...20
Oxygen Administration...20
Suctioning..21
Ventilation Devices..21

Ventilation...21
Mechanics of Ventilation...21
Types of Ventilation...22
Assessment of Ventilation...22
Interventions to Improve Ventilation..22

PATIENT ASSESSMENT...23

Scene Size-up...24

Primary Assessment...25
Initial Impression and General Assessment..25
ABCs: The Lifeline...25
Rapid Medical or Trauma Assessment..25
Priority and Transport Decision...25

History Taking...26
    The Power of Conversation: A Tool in Diagnosis 26
    SAMPLE History: A Systematic Approach...26
    The Importance of Open-Ended Questions 27
    Respecting Patient Privacy 27

Secondary Assessment..27
    The Role of the Secondary Assessment 27
    Components of a Secondary Assessment 27
    A Trauma-Focused Approach...28
    A Medical-Focused Approach...28
    Reassessment 28
    Interpreting the Findings 28

Reassessment 28
    The Significance of Reassessment 28
    How Often Should Reassessment Be Done? 28
    What Does Reassessment Involve? 29
    Documenting Reassessments 29
    The Role of Clinical Judgment 29

MEDICAL EMERGENCIES 31

Respiratory Emergencies...32

Cardiovascular Emergencies 33

Diabetic Emergencies 34

Allergic Reactions..35

Poisoning/Overdose..36

SPECIAL POPULATIONS 39

Obstetrics and Neonatal Care..40

Pediatric Emergencies 41

Geriatric Patients 42

EMS OPERATIONS 45

Ambulance Operations..46

Gaining Access and Patient Extrication 48

Hazardous Materials Incidents 49

Multiple-Casualty Incidents 50

EMS Response to Terrorism...52

PRACTICE TEST 55

Airway Management 55

Patient Assessment 57

Medical Emergencies 59

Trauma 61

Special Populations 63

EMS Operations 65

ANSWER KEY 67

Airway Management 67

Patient Assessment 69

Medical Emergencies... 70

Medical Emergencies... 70

Trauma.. 71

Special Populations 72

EMS Operations... 73

QUESTIONS & ANSWERS 75

Airway Management 75

Patient Assessment 77

Medical emergencies 79

Trauma.. 81

Special Populations 83

EMS Operations... 85

CONCLUSION... 87

SPECIAL EXTRA CONTENT 89

INTRODUCTION

Welcome to this comprehensive Emergency Medical Technician (EMT) exam preparation guide. Our mission is to help aspiring emergency healthcare professionals like you easily navigate the rigorous examination process, boosting your confidence and preparing you to excel. As an EMT, you're at the frontline of medical care, tending to people in their most vulnerable moments. These critical situations demand precision, quick thinking, and in-depth knowledge of emergency medical care. The journey to becoming an EMT, however, is challenging.

One of these is the EMT exam, a pivotal step that requires medical knowledge and the ability to apply it under pressure. This guide is designed to equip you with all the tools you need to pass your EMT exam with flying colors and commence your journey in this challenging yet rewarding field.

The EMT exam may seem daunting, but you're already one step ahead with this guide. Here, you'll find an in-depth review of critical concepts, study strategies that have been tried and tested, practice questions that reflect what you'll face in the actual exam, and guidance on handling the stress that can accompany such a significant test.

This guide is not merely a repository of information; it's an interactive learning resource. The most effective learning happens when active, engaging, and reflective. As such, we have designed this guide to involve you, challenge you, and ultimately build your confidence as you master the skills and knowledge necessary to pass the EMT exam.

We've made it our mission to make your preparation journey smoother. This guide has been carefully crafted to provide clear, concise, and practical information, combining essential medical terminology, emergency care techniques, and professional insights. We've left no stone unturned in our aim to present you with a reliable study resource to illuminate the path to your EMT certification.

So, buckle up for a comprehensive, human, and engaging study journey. Let's conquer the EMT exam together! Your career in emergency medical care awaits. As you set out to become a certified Emergency Medical Technician, the National Registry of Emergency Medical Technicians (NREMT) exam is a formidable milestone. This certification examination is more than just a test—it is a validation of your knowledge, skills, and readiness to serve in real-world medical emergencies.

The NREMT exam is more complex than a simple recall of information. Instead, it's a comprehensive assessment designed to measure your understanding and application of critical concepts, patient assessment, and management in emergency care. The Cognitive Exam is a computer adaptive test (CAT). These queries span various emergency care domains, including airway, respiration, and ventilation; cardiology and resuscitation; trauma; medical and obstetrics/gynecology; and EMS operations. You'll have two hours to complete this portion of the test.

To better prepare you for what lies ahead, this guide will delve deeper into each component of the NREMT exam, offering detailed insights into the subject matter, practical tips, and strategies to tackle each section effectively. Remember, the NREMT exam is not just about book smarts—it's about applying your knowledge and skills in high-stakes, high-pressure situations. This guide is designed to help you meet the exam's demands and ultimately thrive in your role as a certified EMT.

Approaching the NREMT exam can be intimidating, but armed with determination, the right resources, and thorough preparation; you can conquer this challenge. You're not just studying for a test but gearing up for a rewarding, impactful career in emergency medical services. Let's walk this path together!

PREPARATORY

Welcome to the foundational stage of your journey to conquer the NREMT Cognitive exam— the preparatory phase. This critical first step will arm you with the necessary knowledge and tools for your EMT examination, laying down a solid base upon which you will build your understanding of emergency medical care.

To navigate the intricate labyrinth of EMT knowledge, you need to understand how it's structured. The NREMT Cognitive exam covers five key domains: Airway, Respiration, and Ventilation; Cardiology and Resuscitation; Trauma; Medical and Obstetrics/Gynecology; and EMS Operations. Our preparatory chapter will briefly introduce these domains, highlighting critical focus areas. This will not only help you get a feel for what's coming but also enable you to formulate an effective study plan.

First, the Airway, Respiration, and Ventilation domain explores the essentials of maintaining a patient's airway and ensuring adequate respiration and ventilation. Here, you'll delve into subjects such as anatomy and physiology of the respiratory system, respiratory emergencies, airway management techniques, and ventilation devices. You'll learn how to assess a patient's airway, identify potential issues, and employ life-saving procedures to secure the airway and support breathing. Next, Cardiology and Resuscitation focuses on the cardiovascular system and the vital skills required in cardiac arrest scenarios. You'll learn about heart anatomy, electrocardiography (ECG) principles, cardiac emergencies, and resuscitation techniques. Understanding the heart's functions and potential malfunctions is crucial, as heart-related emergencies are common in pre-hospital care.

The Trauma domain delves into assessing and managing various trauma cases, including head, spinal, thoracic, abdominal, and extremity trauma. Trauma care is a cornerstone of emergency medical services, so a sound knowledge of injury mechanisms, assessment strategies, and management principles is vital for every EMT. The Medical and Obstetrics/Gynecology domain spans various medical conditions and emergencies, including neurological, gastrointestinal, genitourinary, and endocrine emergencies. It also covers the fundamentals of obstetric and gynecological emergencies. This broad category prepares you for the field's vast medical scenarios.

Finally, the EMS Operations domain is about understanding the broader emergency services system, including incident command, patient transport, communication, and safety. This knowledge is crucial for efficient and effective operation within an EMS system.

As you begin to study, remember that understanding and memorizing are different. The NREMT exam isn't just about what you know but how you apply that knowledge. Strive to understand concepts deeper, focusing on the 'why' as much as the 'what.' This deeper comprehension will serve you well when asked to apply knowledge to patient scenarios.

Developing a study plan is another crucial step in your preparation. A well-thought-out plan will keep you focused, organized, and motivated. Identify the areas that need the most attention, allocate study time appropriately, and remember to include regular breaks for rest and rejuvenation. Preparation for the NREMT exam isn't just about hitting the books—it's also about taking care of your physical and mental health. Regular exercise, a balanced diet, and adequate sleep can significantly enhance cognitive function and stamina. In conclusion, this preparatory phase allows you to set the stage for success.

You're building the foundation upon which your EMT career will stand. As you embark on this learning journey, remember to be patient with yourself, remain focused, and celebrate your progress. Let's dive into the fascinating world of emergency medical care and take the first step towards mastering your NREMT Cognitive exam!

EMS Systems

The Emergency Medical Services (EMS) System plays a pivotal role in emergency healthcare. It is the life-saving backbone of our healthcare system, designed to respond swiftly and efficiently to medical emergencies. Understanding the structure and function of the EMS system is critical for any aspiring Emergency Medical Technician.

The EMS system encompasses a broad spectrum of services and organizations working in unison to ensure that the response is swift, coordinated, and effective when an emergency strikes. The system comprises multiple components, each performing a specific function. However, despite their roles, they all share a common goal: providing timely, high-quality care to emergency patients.

One of the initial elements of the EMS system is Emergency Medical Dispatch (EMD). This component is often the first point of contact in an emergency scenario. When a member of the public dials an emergency number, trained EMD professionals receive the call. Their responsibilities involve assessing the situation, providing immediate telephonic guidance, and mobilizing the appropriate resources.

Emergency medical technicians and paramedics form the 'first response' layer of the EMS system. These highly trained professionals are dispatched to the emergency scene for immediate medical care. They assess patients, administer life-saving interventions, and determine the most appropriate healthcare facility for their needs.

Another significant element of the EMS system is the ambulance service. This component is responsible for the safe and efficient transport of patients to healthcare facilities. It is important to note that the role of ambulance services extends beyond mere transportation. Ambulances are often 'mobile treatment units,' where EMTs and paramedics continue to provide essential medical care during transit.

The hospital emergency department (ED) forms the following link in the EMS chain. ED professionals, including doctors, nurses, and other healthcare staff, take over patient care upon arrival. The ED staff works closely with the EMTs and paramedics to understand the patient's condition and the treatments administered on route. This collaboration ensures continuity of care.

Post-hospital care and rehabilitation services are also crucial to the EMS system. These services are responsible for the patient's recovery and rehabilitation following an emergency. Depending on the patient's needs, they include home healthcare providers, physical therapists, occupational therapists, and other specialists.

As an aspiring EMT, it's essential to understand your role within this vast and complex system. Not only does it help you see the bigger picture of emergency care, but it also underlines the importance of your function within it. The EMS system is like a well-oiled machine; as an EMT, you're a vital cog. You should also be aware of the legal and ethical aspects of the EMS system. As an EMT, you'll have a legal and moral duty to provide the best possible care to your patients. This involves understanding the principles of medical law and ethics, including patient consent, confidentiality, and the duty to treat.

A thorough understanding of the EMS system will also help you comprehend the importance of communication in emergency care. The EMS system is a team effort. Clear, accurate communication within your immediate team and with other system components is vital to ensure effective patient care.

The EMS system is a complex, multifaceted entity designed to deliver high-quality emergency care to those in need. As an EMT, your role within this system is significant. Your actions can directly impact patient outcomes, making your understanding of the EMS system, your role, and navigating it essential. Remember, as an EMT, you're not just a healthcare provider but a vital part of a life-saving system. Becoming an EMT is about more than just acquiring knowledge and skills. It's about understanding where you fit into the larger picture and how your role contributes to the greater good. You're becoming a part of something bigger than yourself—a system that saves lives daily.

Safety and Well-being of the EMT

In the high-intensity field of emergency medical services, where lives are often on the line, the safety and well-being of Emergency Medical Technicians (EMTs) are paramount. EMTs are the frontline warriors of healthcare, and their welfare is integral not only for their health but also for the overall effectiveness of the emergency response system.

Physical Safety

The physical safety of an EMT is grounded in a strong understanding and adherence to safety protocols and procedures. Every detail matters, from proper lifting techniques to protect against back injuries to using Personal Protective Equipment (PPE) to minimize exposure to infectious diseases. The job often requires handling heavy equipment, maneuvering tight spaces, and dealing with unpredictable scenarios. Training in body mechanics and proper equipment use is not just advisable; it's a necessity.

Emotional Well-being

The emotional toll on EMTs can be as taxing as the job's physical demands. Regular exposure to traumatic situations, life-and-death decisions, and the natural emotional investment in patients can lead to stress and burnout. Emotional well-being is often overlooked but is as critical as physical safety. Support systems, debriefing sessions, and mental health resources should be in place to help EMTs process their experiences and emotions.

Professional Conduct and Ethics

An EMT's professional conduct is vital to their safety and well-being. Adherence to ethical guidelines, including patient confidentiality, informed consent, and non-discrimination, safeguards the integrity of the profession and the individual EMT. Understanding and respecting these principles is essential.

Fitness and Health

EMTs must be physically and mentally healthy to perform their duties effectively. This means maintaining a fitness regimen, eating a balanced diet, and ensuring adequate rest. Regular medical check-ups and vaccinations are also part of maintaining optimum health.

Ongoing Education and Training

The landscape of emergency medical care is continually evolving. Keeping abreast of new technologies, methodologies, and best practices is vital for an EMT's safety and efficacy. Ongoing education and training foster a culture of continuous improvement and adaptation.

Crisis and Fatigue Management

Dealing with long shifts, unpredictable hours, and intense situations can lead to fatigue and burnout. Understanding how to manage fatigue through proper scheduling, rest, and support is essential for the long-term well-being of an EMT. The role of an EMT is complex and demanding, requiring a multifaceted approach to ensure their safety and well-being. The intricate balance of physical security, emotional well-being, professional conduct, personal health, continuous education, and fatigue management shapes a resilient and competent EMT.

Understanding these aspects is vital for individual EMTs and the EMS system's overall effectiveness. A well-cared-for EMT is likelier to perform efficiently, make sound judgments, and provide high-quality patient care. Therefore, the safety and well-being of EMTs are not just personal concerns; they are professional imperatives. In the fast-paced world of emergency medical care, where every second counts, an EMT's physical and mental readiness can mean the difference between life and death. It's a responsibility beyond the self, impacting patients, families, communities, and the entire EMS system. Therefore, the investment in the safety and well-being of EMTs is an investment in the health and resilience of our whole society.

Medical, Legal, and Ethical Issues

As an Emergency Medical Technician (EMT), you're a crucial link between the patient and the emergency medical system. This role carries a significant level of responsibility, and the actions you take (or don't take) can have substantial legal and ethical implications. A comprehensive understanding of the medical, legal, and moral landscape is critical for performing your duties effectively and responsibly.

Medical Issues

Medical issues can range from accurately assessing a patient's condition to deciding the best course of action under time pressure. EMTs must apply their medical knowledge, training, and judgment to provide the appropriate standard of care. However, it's equally important to recognize the limits of your expertise and when it's necessary to call for more advanced medical help.

Legal Issues

Legal issues in emergency medical services primarily revolve around the concept of "duty to act," "consent," and "negligence."

"Duty to act" refers to your legal obligation as an EMT to provide emergency care. Once the patient care process has started, you must continue giving care until transferring the patient to someone with equal or higher medical training is safe.

"Consent" means obtaining permission from the patient to provide care. This can be "expressed" (the patient verbally or non-verbally agrees to receive care) or "implied" (the patient is unconscious or unable to make an informed decision, and it's reasonable to assume they would want care). In the case of minors, consent must generally be obtained from a parent or guardian, except in life-threatening situations.

"Negligence" refers to a failure to act or act outside the acceptable standard of care, resulting in harm to the patient. As an EMT, it's your legal responsibility to provide care that meets a certain standard. This standard could result in legal consequences.

Ethical Issues

While legal issues focus on laws and regulations, ethical issues pertain to moral principles and values. Ethical issues can arise in various scenarios, such as managing a patient who refuses care, dealing with end-of-life decisions, or handling sensitive information.

As an EMT, you must uphold ethical standards like patient autonomy, beneficence (doing good), non-maleficence (avoiding harm), and justice (fairness and equality). Respect for patient autonomy means acknowledging and respecting a patient's rights and decisions about their care. Beneficence and non-maleficence involve providing care that benefits the patient and avoids causing harm. Justice implies equal and fair treatment to all patients, regardless of their background or circumstances.

Moreover, confidentiality is another significant ethical concern. EMTs often have access to sensitive patient information, and it's essential to respect and protect this information to maintain patient trust and comply with laws such as the Health Insurance Portability and Accountability Act (HIPAA). In conclusion, navigating the complex terrain of medical, legal, and ethical issues is essential to an EMT's job. A comprehensive understanding of these issues helps EMTs make informed decisions, provide high-quality care, and protect themselves from legal complications. As an EMT, you're a healthcare provider and an advocate for your patients, upholding their rights and dignity while delivering life-saving care. Understanding and effectively managing these issues is vital for your patients' health and your profession's integrity.

The Human Body

A deep understanding of the human body, its intricate systems, and how they interact is essential for an Emergency Medical Technician (EMT). When responding to an emergency, human anatomy and physiology knowledge will guide your patient assessment, dictate your treatment approach, and ultimately influence the outcome.

The Cardiovascular System

The cardiovascular system, often considered the body's lifeblood, is pivotal in maintaining homeostasis. The heart, consisting of four chambers – two atria and two ventricles – contracts and relaxes rhythmically to pump oxygenated blood to the body via arteries and retrieve deoxygenated blood through veins. The smallest blood vessels, capillaries, serve as exchange points for oxygen, nutrients, and waste materials with the body's cells. Understanding the cardiovascular system's function is vital in recognizing signs of life-threatening emergencies, such as myocardial infarctions (heart attacks), congestive heart failure, and various arrhythmias.

The Respiratory System

The respiratory system is designed to inhale oxygen-rich air and exhale carbon dioxide-filled air, a waste product of cellular metabolism. This process starts when we inhale air through our nose or mouth, then travels down the trachea into bronchi, bronchioles, and finally to tiny alveoli in the lungs, where gas exchange occurs. Understanding how the respiratory system functions can help EMTs identify and respond to emergencies, such as COPD (Chronic Obstructive Pulmonary Disease), asthma attacks, and respiratory failure due to trauma or infection.

The Nervous System

The nervous system acts as the body's control center and communication network. It primarily comprises two parts: the central nervous system (CNS), which includes the brain and spinal cord, and the peripheral nervous system, which consists of all the nerves branching off the CNS. The nervous system operates through electrical signals called action potentials, enabling swift communication between various body parts. Understanding this intricate system is crucial for EMTs in responding to neurological emergencies such as stroke, seizures, and traumatic injuries.

The Musculoskeletal System

The musculoskeletal system comprises bones, muscles, cartilage, tendons, ligaments, joints, and other connective tissue. It supports the body, allows movement, and protects vital organs. For example, the rib cage protects the heart and lungs, while the skull protects the brain. EMTs must understand this system to adequately respond to trauma, assess injury severity, apply splints, or immobilize a patient for transport.

The Digestive System

The digestive system is responsible for processing food into usable nutrients for the body. It includes the mouth, esophagus, stomach, small and large intestines, and accessory organs like the liver, gallbladder, and pancreas. The liver, in particular, has multiple functions, including detoxifying harmful substances and metabolizing drugs. Knowledge of this system is essential for EMTs dealing with emergencies like gastrointestinal bleeding, abdominal pain, or suspected poisoning.

The Integumentary System

The integumentary system, including the skin, hair, nails, sweat, and oil glands, acts as the body's first defense against external threats. It helps regulate body temperature and permits touch, heat, and cold sensations. EMTs often deal with integumentary system-related issues, such as burns, lacerations, puncture wounds, and skin infections, making knowledge of this system fundamental.

The Endocrine System

The endocrine system comprises a series of glands that produce and secrete hormones to regulate many body functions, including metabolism, growth and development, tissue function, and mood. The endocrine system's glands include the pituitary, thyroid, parathyroid, adrenal glands, pancreas, and gonads (ovaries and testes). Recognizing emergencies related to this system, like diabetic ketoacidosis or Addisonian crisis, forms a significant part of an EMT's role.

Remember, as an EMT, you won't just face individual system problems; you'll often encounter situations where multiple systems are affected. Understanding how these systems interact will provide a more holistic approach to emergency care and contribute to better patient outcomes.

AIRWAY MANAGEMENT

I n emergency medical services, a foundational principle that drives every action and decision is *"Airway comes first."* As an Emergency Medical Technician (EMT), you must ensure that your patient's airway is open and they can breathe effectively; without this, all other medical interventions would be in vain.

Every breath a person takes involves a complex, finely-tuned series of events. Air, carrying life-sustaining oxygen, enters through the nose or mouth, travels down the pharynx, passes the larynx, and follows the trachea until it reaches the bronchi, which further branch out into smaller tubes and lead to the lungs. In the lungs' tiny air sacs, the alveoli, oxygen transfers into the bloodstream, and carbon dioxide, a waste product, moves from the blood into the lungs to be exhaled. This process, known as gas exchange, is vital to life.

However, this fragile system can be compromised in many ways. Trauma, medical conditions, foreign objects, or unconsciousness can obstruct the airway, hinder breathing, or stop it altogether. In these circumstances, quick, decisive actions by an EMT can make the difference between life and death.

Airway Assessment

The first step in airway management is a thorough airway assessment. Listen, look, and feel for the signs of a patent (open) airway and adequate breathing. Is the patient speaking? Are they gasping for air or making unusual noises like wheezing or gurgling? Do you see chest rise and fall? Is their breathing rate, rhythm, and depth within normal limits?

Basic Airway Maneuvers

You must intervene quickly if the patient's airway is obstructed or their breathing is inadequate. Basic airway maneuvers, such as the head-tilt-chin-lift and jaw-thrust maneuvers, can help open the airway in an unconscious or semi-conscious patient. However, if a spinal injury is suspected, use the jaw-thrust maneuver to avoid moving the neck and potentially causing further damage.

Airway Adjuncts

If basic maneuvers are insufficient, EMTs can use airway adjuncts. Oropharyngeal airways (OPAs) and nasopharyngeal airways (NPAs) can help keep the airway open. Remember, using these devices requires training and practice to ensure correct sizing, insertion, and maintenance.

Suctioning

In cases where the airway is obstructed by fluids such as vomit, blood, or saliva, suctioning may be necessary. A portable suction device can remove these obstructions and help maintain a patent airway.

Oxygen Therapy

Once the airway is clear, the next step is to ensure the patient has adequate oxygen. Depending on the patient's needs, oxygen can be administered through different devices, ranging from nasal cannulas to non-rebreather masks. Monitoring the patient's oxygen saturation with a pulse oximeter can provide a guide to the effectiveness of your interventions.

Ventilation Support

In severe cases where the patient is not breathing effectively, you may need to provide ventilation support. Bag-valve masks (BVMs) can deliver oxygen-rich air to the patient through passive ventilation or an additional oxygen supply.

In summary, airway management is a critical skill for an EMT. Remember the ABCs—Airway, Breathing, and Circulation—your patient's life may depend on them. Continually assess and manage the airway first before moving on to other interventions. Through thorough training and consistent practice, you can master these essential skills and be prepared to face any airway emergency that comes your way.

Airway Anatomy and Physiology

Understanding the complex anatomy and physiology of the human airway is crucial for anyone involved in emergency medical services. By thoroughly knowing how the airway is structured and how it functions, you'll be equipped to handle airway emergencies effectively and confidently. This section will guide you through the intricacies of the human airway, shedding light on its anatomy and the physiological processes it governs.

The airway comprises the upper and lower respiratory tracts. The upper respiratory tract starts at the nostrils and mouth and extends to the vocal cords. The lower respiratory tract spans from the vocal lines down to the alveoli, the tiny air sacs where gas exchange occurs in the lungs. Let's delve deeper into each component.

Upper Airway Anatomy

The upper airway functions to warm, filter, and moisten the air. It consists of:

Nasal Cavity:

- **Structure:** Separated into two passages by the nasal septum, lined with mucous membranes.
- **Function:** Filters dust and pathogens through cilia; warms and moistens the air.

Oral Cavity:

- **Structure:** Includes the lips, teeth, gums, and tongue.
- **Function:** Secondary pathway for breathing, particularly during strenuous activity.

Pharynx:

- **Nasopharynx:** Behind the nasal cavity, lined with ciliated mucosa, connects to the eustachian tubes.
- **Oropharynx:** Includes the soft palate and the tongue base and guides air from the oral cavity into the laryngopharynx.
- **Laryngopharynx:** Connects to the larynx and esophagus, directing food and air into their respective passages.

Larynx:

- **Structure:** Cartilaginous structure housing the vocal cords, protected by the thyroid cartilage (Adam's apple).
- **Function:** Sound production and protection of the trachea from food aspiration.

Lower Airway Anatomy

The lower airway conducts air to the lungs and is made up of:

Trachea:
- **Structure:** Tubular structure made of C-shaped cartilaginous rings.
- **Function:** Conducts air to the lungs.

Bronchi and Bronchioles:
- **Structure:** Branching system of tubes of diminishing size.
- **Function:** Facilitates air movement to and from alveoli.

Lungs and Alveoli:
- **Structure:** Two lungs housing millions of alveoli, tiny sacs surrounded by blood vessels.
- **Function:** Gas exchange – oxygen enters the blood, and carbon dioxide is expelled.

Airway Physiology
The functioning of the airway is a complex process encompassing several vital aspects:

Ventilation:
- **Inhalation:** Diaphragm contracts, lowering the pressure in the lungs and allowing air to flow in.
- **Exhalation:** Diaphragm relaxes, increasing pressure in the lungs, forcing air out.
- **Regulation:** Controlled by the respiratory center in the brainstem, responding to levels of carbon dioxide in the blood.

Gas Exchange:
- **Oxygen Transport:** Oxygen diffuses from the alveoli into the blood, binds to hemoglobin in red blood cells, and is transported to body tissues.
- **Carbon Dioxide Removal:** Carbon dioxide moves from the blood to the alveoli, carried partly as bicarbonate in the plasma, to be exhaled.

Respiratory Defense Mechanisms:
- **Cilia and Mucus:** Trap and remove inhaled foreign particles.
- **Cough Reflex:** Expels foreign substances or irritants.
- **Alveolar Macrophages:** Engulf and digest pathogens within the alveoli.

The airway's structure and functions are intricately related, contributing to essential life-sustaining processes. Understanding these aspects is critical for EMTs in providing adequate care, especially during emergencies involving the airway. Knowledge of airway anatomy and physiology also lays the foundation for the more specialized skills required in airway management techniques, reinforcing the importance of this topic in the EMT exam.

Basic Airway Management

Airway management forms a cornerstone of pre-hospital emergency care, and understanding essential airway management is paramount for every EMT. The objective here is maintaining a patent (open and unblocked) airway, ensuring oxygen delivery to the lungs, and facilitating carbon dioxide removal.

Patient Positioning

Patient positioning is often the first step in managing the airway. EMTs commonly use the "sniffing position" or "head-tilt chin-lift" technique for conscious patients and the "jaw-thrust maneuver" for unconscious patients to maintain airway patency.

- **Sniffing Position:** The patient is placed on their back with the head slightly extended and elevated. This alignment opens the airway and allows for adequate ventilation.

- **Head-Tilt Chin-Lift:** This technique is used for patients without a suspected neck or spine injury. It involves tilting the patient's head back while lifting the chin, which opens the airway.

- **Jaw-Thrust Maneuver:** Ideal for trauma patients where spinal injury is a concern. It involves reaching around the patient's head, grasping the angles of the lower jaw, and lifting with both hands to open the airway without moving the neck.

Manual Airway Techniques and Devices

When positioning isn't enough, EMTs use manual maneuvers and airway adjuncts to ensure patency.

- **Manual Maneuvers:** Manual maneuvers, such as the chin-lift and jaw-thrust, often accompany airway positioning. These maneuvers help to open the airway by moving the tongue away from the back of the throat.

- **Oropharyngeal Airways (OPAs):** OPAs are devices inserted into the mouth to prevent the tongue from blocking the throat. They're used for patients with altered levels of consciousness.

- **Nasopharyngeal Airways (NPAs):** NPAs are inserted through the nostril and rest in the back of the throat, providing an airway route. They're better suited for semi-conscious or conscious patients with a gag reflex.

Oxygen Administration

Supplemental oxygen can be life-saving in many emergencies, helping to maintain adequate oxygen levels in the bloodstream. Oxygen can be administered through various means:

- **Nasal Cannula:** This device is well tolerated and delivers low oxygen concentrations. It is suitable for patients requiring minimal oxygen supplementation.

- **Simple Face Mask:** This mask covers the patient's nose and mouth and can deliver moderate oxygen concentrations. It is used when higher oxygen delivery is necessary.

- **Non-rebreather Mask (NRM):** This mask provides the highest oxygen concentration and is used in severe cases, such as shock or significant difficulty in breathing.

Suctioning

Suctioning is a crucial procedure used when there is an obstruction in the airway due to fluids such as vomit, blood, or secretions. The process involves using a suction device with a rigid suction catheter (also known as a "tonsil tip") or a flexible suction catheter.

- **Rigid Suction Catheter:** These are used primarily for suctioning the mouth, where they can effectively remove larger pieces of debris.

- **Flexible Suction Catheter:** These are more suited for suctioning the nose or when the patient's mouth can't open widely.

Regardless of the patient's condition, the suctioning process should never take longer than 15 seconds, as extended suctioning can lead to hypoxia.

Ventilation Devices

When patients are unable to ventilate adequately on their own, EMTs may need to employ mechanical ventilation. Bag-valve masks (BVMs) are commonly used for this purpose.

- **Bag-Valve Masks (BVMs):** BVMs are handheld devices used to provide positive pressure ventilation to patients who are not breathing or not breathing adequately. BVMs can be used with or without supplemental oxygen.

Remember, essential airway management is the critical first step in patient care and often sets the tone for all further interventions. This basic knowledge is a foundation for more advanced airway management techniques, emphasizing the importance of this topic in the EMT exam.

Ventilation

Ventilation is a pivotal element of emergency care and the EMT exam. Simply put, ventilation is the process by which oxygen-enriched air flows into the lungs, and waste gases like carbon dioxide are expelled. Ventilation forms the second step of the airway management pyramid after ensuring a patent airway. Now, let's break down its aspects to aid your understanding.

Mechanics of Ventilation

Ventilation is an intricate physiological process, the understanding of which is vital for an EMT—the respiratory system, comprising the lungs and air passages, functions as a mechanical system.

During inhalation, the diaphragm and external intercostal muscles contract, increasing the chest cavity's size. This expansion lowers the pressure within the lungs, drawing air into them. Conversely, these muscles relax during exhalation, decreasing the chest cavity's size. The pressure within the lungs rises, forcing air out.

Ventilation can be voluntary, controlled by the cerebral cortex, or involuntary, regulated by the medulla oblongata in response to the blood's carbon dioxide and oxygen levels. The balance between oxygen intake and carbon dioxide removal is pivotal for the body's homeostasis.

Types of Ventilation

There are two principal types of ventilation: spontaneous and mechanical.

- **Spontaneous ventilation** refers to the patient's ability to ventilate without external assistance. Assessment of spontaneous ventilation includes observing the rate, depth, and quality of the patient's breathing.

- **Mechanical ventilation** uses external devices, like a bag-valve-mask (BVM) or an automatic transport ventilator, to assist or control the patient's ventilation. Mechanical ventilation becomes necessary when a patient cannot maintain adequate spontaneous ventilation.

Assessment of Ventilation

Assessing a patient's ventilation is crucial in determining if intervention is necessary. EMTs primarily rely on visual cues, such as chest rise and fall, use of accessory muscles, and skin color. Auditory cues, like the sound of breathing, can also be important. Monitoring devices, like pulse oximetry and capnography, can objectively measure a patient's ventilation status.

Interventions to Improve Ventilation

When a patient's spontaneous ventilation is inadequate, interventions become necessary. This may involve using adjuncts to maintain an open airway, providing supplemental oxygen, or mechanically ventilating the patient.

- **Airway Adjuncts:** These can help maintain an open airway, improving ventilation. The type of adjunct used, whether an oropharyngeal or nasopharyngeal airway, will depend on the patient's level of consciousness and potential for a gag reflex.

- **Supplemental Oxygen:** Supplemental oxygen can improve the oxygen content of the blood, improving the effectiveness of each breath. The method used to deliver supplemental oxygen can vary based on the patient's condition.

- **Mechanical Ventilation:** If a patient cannot ventilate adequately, EMTs may need to provide ventilation. This can involve using a bag-valve mask or an automatic transport ventilator.

Ventilation is essential to patient care, and understanding it is crucial for success in the EMT exam. Proficiency in assessing and managing a patient's ventilation can be the difference between life and death in the pre-hospital setting.

PATIENT ASSESSMENT

Patient assessment is a cornerstone of emergency medical care. As an Emergency Medical Technician (EMT), your ability to assess a patient accurately and promptly is not only a skill tested on the National Registry of Emergency Medical Technicians (NREMT) exam but a vital ability you will rely on in real-world situations. Patient assessment involves steps and considerations, each as crucial as the next, which form the bedrock of efficient and effective pre-hospital care.

A systematic, comprehensive approach to patient assessment enables EMTs to identify and prioritize a patient's needs based on their condition. This process begins when you approach the scene and continues until the patient is transferred to definitive care. Understanding each phase of this procedure is critical, as each informs the subsequent steps and therapeutic decisions.

At the core of patient assessment is "no harm." This tenet underscores the necessity of an EMT's ability to gather data without causing physical or psychological injury to the patient. A skillful EMT considers their approach to the patient, respecting boundaries and maintaining professionalism without jeopardizing the assessment's efficiency.

The initial impression of the patient forms the beginning of the assessment. As EMTs, your approach to the scene, safety measures, and how you make your presence known to the patient can significantly influence the outcome of the patient's situation. Making a rapid scan of the patient from head to toe can provide valuable insights into their status. Identifying life-threatening conditions is the priority during this stage, and recognizing these quickly can make the difference between life and death.

Following the initial impression, the EMT performs a systematic assessment, moving through a specific sequence of steps. This typically includes scene safety, mechanism of injury/nature of illness determination, primary survey, history taking, secondary assessment, and reassessment.

The primary survey focuses on assessing the patient's airway, breathing, and circulation - often remembered by the ABC acronym. Any life-threatening problems identified during this survey should be immediately managed.

During history taking, the EMT seeks better to understand the patient's symptoms and medical history. Here, EMTs often use the SAMPLE acronym to recall the key elements to ask: Symptoms, Allergies, Medications, Past medical history, Last oral intake, and Events leading up to the present illness or injury.

The secondary assessment involves a more detailed examination of the patient. This step may involve a head-to-toe physical exam, focused exams depending on the patient's complaints, and ongoing monitoring of vital signs.

Regular reassessments are performed to identify patient condition changes over time. These reassessments are crucial as they inform any changes in the patient's management that may be required.

Understanding and mastering the patient assessment process is critical to successful EMTs. Remember, the goal of patient assessment is not just to pass your NREMT exam but to provide the highest quality of care to your patients in the field. Keep this objective in mind as you prepare, and you will undoubtedly achieve success both on the test and in your career.

Scene Size-up

A crucial aspect of patient assessment that every aspiring EMT needs to be proficient at is the scene size-up. The scene size-up is the first step in any emergency and sets the foundation for the following actions. This is where you, as an EMT, must look, listen, and feel to understand the scene's dynamics you are stepping into. Let's delve into the significance of the scene size-up, its components, and how mastering this skill can augment patient care.

Scene size-up begins even before you step foot at the scene. It starts the moment you receive the dispatch information. That initial information will shape your mindset and help you formulate a plan of action. As you approach the scene, observing your surroundings and noting anything unusual is essential. This could be anything from the behavior of bystanders to the position of a vehicle involved in an accident. These observations can provide vital clues about what happened and the possible injuries the patient might have sustained.

One of the first things to consider in the scene size-up is safety. Is the scene safe for you, your team, the patient, and any bystanders? This step is more complex than it might sound. Hazards could be apparent, like a fire, or subtle, like a potential domestic violence situation. If the scene is unsafe, you should await additional resources to mitigate the hazards before proceeding. Remember, an injured or incapacitated EMT can't help anyone. In your role as an EMT, your safety is paramount.

Next, consider the mechanism of injury or the nature of the illness. What has caused the emergency? A fall from a height may have caused trauma, or a known cardiac patient may be suffering from chest pain. Identifying the probable cause can guide your treatment and inform the urgency of your actions.

Now, let's talk about the number of patients. Is there one patient, or are there multiple patients? The number of patients can dictate the resources you need. You may need additional ambulances or even activate a mass casualty incident plan for various patients.

Consider also the need for any additional resources. Depending on the nature of the incident, you may require law enforcement, fire services, or a specialized medical team. Early identification of these needs can expedite their dispatch and arrival, improving the overall response to the incident.

Finally, consider the question - what is your general impression of the patient? Your public image is formed by observing the patient's appearance, body positioning, level of distress, and any visible injuries. This first impression can provide a wealth of information and guide the urgency of your actions.

The scene size-up is a continuous process, not a one-time event. As the situation evolves, so should your assessment. The information gathered during the scene size-up guides the next stages of the patient assessment process, the primary survey and secondary assessments.

Each aspect of the scene size-up is a piece of the puzzle that, when put together, creates a clear picture of the incident. Every piece of information, no matter how small, can significantly impact patient outcomes.

Therefore, developing a keen eye and an analytical mind for effective scene size-ups is vital for an EMT. By practicing and mastering this skill, you can enhance the level of care you provide to your patients, which is the ultimate goal of any healthcare professional. Remember, the scene size-up isn't just a checklist to be completed; it's the foundation upon which life-saving decisions are made.

Primary Assessment

Embarking on the pivotal aspect of patient evaluation, the primary assessment, it is essential to understand its significance and execution in Emergency Medical Services (EMS). Upon completing the scene size-up, your attention must swiftly shift to your patient, requiring a rapid yet thorough assessment. The primary evaluation entails a systematic approach to quickly identifying and managing immediate life threats.

Initial Impression and General Assessment

At the beginning of the primary assessment, the initial impression plays a critical role. This impression is formed based on your overall perception of the patient. What is their level of consciousness? Do they appear comfortable or in distress? Remember, appearances can be deceiving. A patient who initially seems stable could quickly deteriorate without warning. Hence, this initial stage demands a keen observational skill, where each detail contributes to painting a complete picture of the patient's status.

ABCs: The Lifeline

Emerging from the initial impression, you arrive at the crux of primary assessment - **ABC: Airway, Breathing, and Circulation.** Each component is not merely an individual aspect but a critical lifeline determining the patient's immediate condition. The airway is your first priority. A blocked airway can quickly lead to hypoxia and cardiac arrest. Look, listen, and feel for signs of obstruction or inadequate air movement. Is the patient able to speak? Are there unusual noises like stridor or gurgling? Prompt intervention, such as repositioning or suctioning, may be necessary to clear the airway.

Next, evaluate breathing. Is the patient breathing adequately? Consider the rate, rhythm, depth, and quality of respirations. Use your stethoscope to listen for breath sounds. Are they symmetrical? Are there signs of distress, like cyanosis or the use of accessory muscles? Interventions may include oxygen administration or even manual ventilations. The final component, circulation, demands an assessment of the patient's pulse and skin characteristics. The pulse provides insight into the patient's heart rate and rhythm. Skin color, temperature, and condition (dry, moist, or clammy) can explain circulatory status. Remember to check for severe bleeding, which could directly threaten circulation.

Rapid Medical or Trauma Assessment

Following the ABCs, conduct a focused yet swift examination of the patient's body. This would be a Rapid Medical Assessment for medical patients and a Rapid Trauma Assessment for trauma patients. You're looking for obvious signs of injury or illness that need immediate intervention.

Priority and Transport Decision

The primary assessment concludes with determining patient priority and the decision to transport. Critical or potentially unstable patients should be transported immediately, with a detailed evaluation and interventions performed on route. Stable patients may be thoroughly assessed and treated on the scene before transport. Remember, the primary assessment is dynamic, not static. As an EMT, you must continually re-evaluate your patient, especially if their condition changes or your interventions don't have the expected effect.

Mastering the primary assessment can mean the difference between life and death for your patient. By accurately interpreting the signs and symptoms presented and acting swiftly and appropriately, you have the potential to impact patient outcomes significantly. Therefore, this skill is not just a requisite for the EMT exam but also a cornerstone for your future career in emergency medical services. Practice it, refine it, and you will find that you are an integral part of the chain that saves lives daily.

History Taking

Understanding the importance and technique of history-taking is crucial for every EMT. Amidst the chaos of an emergency scene, it's easy to overlook this vital step. However, during these important moments of interaction with the patient, you gather information critical to their treatment and transport. With a thorough and accurate history, you may notice vital signs of their condition or make correct judgments, potentially leading to appropriate management.

The Power of Conversation: A Tool in Diagnosis

When you engage your patient in conversation, you do more than talk - you are actively collecting data. Information provided by the patient, their family, or bystanders can reveal essential clues about the patient's condition. This can help guide your treatment decisions and provide the hospital with valuable information.

SAMPLE History: A Systematic Approach

One standard method of history taking is the SAMPLE history. This mnemonic acronym stands for **Symptoms, Allergies, Medications, Past Medical History, Last Oral Intake, and Events Leading Up to Present Illness**. Each component serves to guide you through an organized, methodical process of questioning.

- **Symptoms** are the patient's complaints, described in their own words. Understanding the symptomatology helps create a clinical picture. Is the patient experiencing chest pain? Difficulty breathing? Each symptom paints a piece of the larger image.

- **Allergies** can be critical when deciding on treatment options. If a patient is allergic to a medication you are considering, this could lead to a potentially severe allergic reaction.

- **Medications** are another crucial element. What prescriptions does the patient currently take? Are they on blood thinners, which could impact bleeding? Have they missed a dose of a crucial medication?

- **Past Medical History** can reveal potential complications or underlying conditions that can impact the current illness or injury. For instance, a patient with a history of heart disease may be more prone to cardiac-related complications.

- **Last Oral Intake** refers to the last thing the patient ate or drank. This information can be vital in cases of abdominal pain or when anesthesia may be required at the hospital.

- **Events Leading Up to Present Illness** allow you to understand the context and potential triggers for the current situation. Did the chest pain begin after a heated argument or during physical activity?

Remember, the SAMPLE history is not a rigid protocol; it's a guide. Adapt it as needed based on the patient's condition and your judgment as an EMT.

The Importance of Open-Ended Questions

While taking a history, remember to ask open-ended questions that encourage the patient to provide detailed responses. Instead of asking, "Did the pain start suddenly?" ask, "Can you tell me how the pain started?". This way, you get a more elaborate answer, not just a simple 'yes' or 'no.'

Respecting Patient Privacy

It's important to remember that taking a history is not just a medical process but also an interpersonal one. Patients may feel vulnerable or anxious, especially in an emergency. Always approach the process empathetically, ensuring the patient's comfort and privacy.

In conclusion, history-taking is an indispensable skill for an EMT. It offers a path to a better understanding of the patient's ailment beyond what can be observed from the exterior. By mastering the technique of effective communication and incorporating a systematic approach, like the SAMPLE history, you can ensure you are providing the best possible care for your patients. This skill proves beneficial for the EMT exam and serves as a core component of your career in emergency medical services.

Secondary Assessment

One of the most powerful tools in the EMT's toolkit is the Secondary Assessment. It's a systematic approach that allows EMTs to uncover critical information about a patient's condition. This information might take time to be apparent, but it can heavily influence patient care and transport decisions.

The Role of the Secondary Assessment

Once the primary assessment and history taking are complete and the patient's life threats are managed, EMTs transition to the secondary inspection. Here, the EMT takes a more detailed examination of the patient to identify injuries or conditions that need further medical attention. This assessment aids in forming a differential diagnosis and further refines the treatment plan.

Components of a Secondary Assessment

The secondary assessment comprises two main components: a systematic physical examination and a set of vital signs. This examination should be thorough and efficient, ensuring no potential injuries or conditions are missed. The vitals collected provide quantitative data about the patient's current physiological state.

- **Physical Examination:** The physical examination in the secondary assessment is a head-to-toe survey for a trauma patient and a focused exam for a medical patient. For trauma patients, you methodically examine the patient from head to toe, looking for signs of injury. In contrast, for medical patients, the examination is more focused on the body system or systems that the patient's signs and symptoms suggest may be involved.

- **Vital Signs:** Vital signs are objective measurements of essential body functions and provide information about the patient's overall physiological status. These measurements usually include the patient's pulse, blood pressure, respiratory rate, and SpO2 (blood oxygen saturation). Changes in vital signs over time can provide crucial information about the patient's condition.

A Trauma-Focused Approach

For trauma patients, the secondary assessment involves a systematic head-to-toe examination. You begin at the head, examining the scalp, ears, eyes, nose, and mouth for signs of trauma. Next, you move on to the neck, checking for jugular vein distension or tracheal deviation. This pattern continues down the body, checking each region for deformity, contusions, abrasions, punctures/penetrations, burns, tenderness, lacerations, and swelling (DCAP-BTLS).

A Medical-Focused Approach

In contrast, the secondary assessment is a focused exam for medical patients. The aim is not to examine the whole body, but to focus on a specific system or part of the body, guided by the patient's symptoms and history. For instance, if the patient has difficulty breathing, you would focus on the respiratory system, looking for signs like wheezing, abnormal breath sounds, or cyanosis.

Reassessment

Secondary assessment is a process that is more than just a one-time process. You should regularly reassess your patient, particularly the vital signs and primary assessment components. For an unstable patient, reassessment should occur every 5 minutes; for a stable patient, it should occur every 15 minutes.

Interpreting the Findings

The secondary assessment is about more than just data collection. It's about understanding what the findings mean. As an EMT, you must learn how to interpret and integrate these findings into your ongoing patient care. In conclusion, the secondary assessment is a vital step in patient care, serving as a bridge between the primary evaluation and the ongoing maintenance of the patient. By conducting a thorough secondary assessment, you can ensure you've not missed any injuries or conditions, allowing you to provide the best possible care for your patients. Every piece of information counts in the high-stakes world of emergency medical services, making the secondary assessment an essential skill for both the EMT exam and your professional practice.

Reassessment

In the dynamic environment of emergency medicine, patient conditions can change rapidly, sometimes in the blink of an eye. EMTs must remain ever-vigilant, continuously re-evaluating their patients' needs. This continuous evaluation process, known as reassessment, is an indispensable part of the EMT's workflow.

The Significance of Reassessment

Reassessment is a vital tool in the EMT's arsenal. It enables EMTs to promptly identify changes in the patient's condition, allowing for immediate adjustment of the treatment plan. Regular reassessment is necessary for deteriorations or improvements in the patient's essential to be noticed, leading to delayed interventions or unnecessary treatments.

How Often Should Reassessment Be Done?

The patient's condition primarily determines the frequency of reassessment. Generally, a stable patient should be reassessed every 15 minutes, while an unstable patient requires reassessment every 5 minutes. However, a reassessment should also be performed after every intervention to gauge its effectiveness and identify any potential complications.

What Does Reassessment Involve?

The reassessment process mirrors the primary and secondary assessments on a streamlined scale. It involves repeating the preliminary evaluation, reassessing vital signs, rechecking interventions, and evaluating the patient's response to treatment.

- **Repeating Primary Assessment:** The primary assessment, including assessing the patient's level of consciousness, airway, breathing, and circulation, is quickly repeated to ensure that the patient's status has not changed or deteriorated.

- **Reassessing Vital Signs:** Vital signs, including pulse, blood pressure, respiratory rate, and SpO2, are reassessed to provide objective data on the patient's physiological condition. Any significant changes could indicate an improvement or worsening of the patient's status.

- **Rechecking Interventions:** All interventions performed should be rechecked to ensure they are still correctly in place and functioning as intended. For instance, intravenous lines and splints or bandages should be rechecked for patency for proper positioning and effectiveness.

- **Evaluating Response to Treatment:** Assessing the patient's response to interventions and treatments is a crucial reassessment component. This could involve asking the patient about their pain levels, observing their symptoms, or noting any physiological changes.

Documenting Reassessments

Documentation is a crucial part of the reassessment process. Each reassessment should be thoroughly documented, including the findings and any changes in the patient's condition or treatment plan. Proper documentation helps ensure continuity of care, provides a legal record of the care provided and can aid in future research and quality improvement efforts.

The Role of Clinical Judgment

While guidelines provide a general timeline for reassessment, it's essential to remember that every patient is unique. Therefore, the need for and frequency of reassessment may vary. EMTs should use their clinical judgment and consider factors such as the patient's age, underlying health conditions, nature and severity of injuries or illness, response to treatment, and transport time to the hospital.

In conclusion, reassessment is a powerful tool for maintaining situational awareness and ensuring the highest quality of patient care. It's a dynamic, ongoing process that requires EMTs to be observant, responsive, and adaptable. As an aspiring EMT, developing strong reassessment skills will assist you in acing your EMT exam and set the foundation for your future success in the ever-evolving world of emergency medical services.

MEDICAL EMERGENCIES

Medical emergencies are a significant aspect of the EMT profession. As first responders, EMTs are frequently called upon to provide pre-hospital care to patients suffering from various medical emergencies. These can range from cardiac arrests and strokes to seizures, respiratory distress, diabetic emergencies, and more. Understanding the nature of these emergencies and the appropriate response strategies is crucial to providing effective emergency medical care.

An EMT's role in responding to medical emergencies encompasses rapid assessment, immediate intervention, and transport to definitive care, all while providing comfort and reassurance to the patient. Through a combination of theoretical knowledge and practical skills, EMTs ensure the best possible outcomes for their patients in life-or-death situations.

Cardiovascular emergencies, such as heart attacks and strokes, are among the most common medical emergencies EMTs encounter. Prompt recognition of these conditions, based on symptoms like chest pain, difficulty breathing, and weakness or numbness on one side of the body, is essential. Initial care typically includes administering oxygen, assisting with prescribed medications like nitroglycerin or aspirin, monitoring vital signs, and rapid transport to a hospital.

Respiratory emergencies, including asthma, COPD exacerbation, and pulmonary edema, can also present significant challenges. Difficulty breathing is a common symptom, and immediate intervention is crucial to prevent respiratory failure. EMTs must know how to administer nebulized medications, assist with prescribed inhalers, and provide ventilatory assistance if needed.

Neurological emergencies such as seizures, strokes, and altered mental status require EMTs to see signs and symptoms keenly. These include changes in behavior, coordination, strength, or sensation. Rapid recognition, stabilization of the patient's condition, and transport to an appropriate medical facility are critical aspects of care.

Endocrine emergencies, like diabetic emergencies, demand an understanding of the impact of insulin and glucose on the body. Hypoglycemia (low blood sugar) and hyperglycemia (high blood sugar) can both present life-threatening emergencies. EMTs need to recognize these conditions based on signs like altered mental status, abnormal behavior, and rapid heart rate, then provide appropriate care, including administering glucose or facilitating insulin administration as needed.

It's important to remember that every patient and every emergency is unique. The above situations represent just a fraction of the medical emergencies EMTs may encounter. Others include allergic reactions, overdoses, poisonings, and environmental emergencies like heatstroke or hypothermia. Each situation requires a distinct approach based on the patient's presenting symptoms and the EMT's medical knowledge and skills.

In preparing for your EMT exam, it's essential to gain a comprehensive understanding of the wide variety of medical emergencies you may encounter in the field. This understanding goes beyond simply memorizing symptoms and treatments. It also includes developing the ability to think critically and make swift, informed decisions under pressure – skills that will help you pass your exam and serve you well throughout your career as an EMT.

The chapter on "Medical Emergencies" is dedicated to providing you with the knowledge and tools you'll need to face these challenging situations with confidence. So, let's delve deeper into the world of medical emergencies and arm you with the information you need to provide the best care possible for your future patients.

Respiratory Emergencies

In the landscape of medical emergencies, respiratory distress holds a pivotal position. EMTs frequently respond to calls involving patients struggling to breathe, and each scenario requires a distinct approach informed by a deep understanding of respiratory anatomy, physiology, and pathology.

Recognizing Respiratory Distress

The first step in managing respiratory emergencies is recognizing when a patient is in distress. This might appear straightforward – a person struggling to breathe is hard to miss – but the reality can be more nuanced. Respiratory distress can manifest in various ways, from overt difficulty breathing to more subtle signs like anxiety, restlessness, or changes in mental status. Specific indicators to watch include abnormal respiratory rates (either too fast or too slow), use of accessory muscles for breathing, strange breath sounds, and cyanosis (a bluish skin discoloration of the skin and mucous membranes due to low oxygen levels).

Differentiating Respiratory Conditions

The underlying causes of respiratory distress can be vast, each presenting with unique symptoms and requiring specific interventions. Asthma, for instance, is an inflammatory disease leading to constriction of the airways. Patients with an asthma attack might present with wheezing, coughing, chest tightness, and increased respiratory effort. In contrast, Chronic Obstructive Pulmonary Disease (COPD) involves progressive damage to the airways and lungs, leading to shortness of breath, productive cough, and frequent respiratory infections.

Pulmonary edema, often resulting from congestive heart failure, presents shortness of breath, especially when lying flat (orthopnea), and wet, productive cough, often with pink, frothy sputum. Finally, patients with pneumonia might show signs of infection like fever and chills, productive cough, chest pain, and possibly altered breath sounds on one side of the chest.

Initial Management Strategies

Regardless of the underlying cause, initial management of respiratory distress involves ensuring an open airway, providing supplemental oxygen, and assessing vital signs, including pulse oximetry. In many cases, simply positioning the patient upright can improve breathing. Assisted ventilation may be required in severe cases.

Specific Interventions

Beyond these general measures, specific interventions depend on the underlying cause; for asthma and COPD, bronchodilators – medications that relax the muscles around the airways – can be administered, often in the form of metered-dose inhalers or nebulized treatments. In cases of pulmonary edema, nitroglycerin, and continuous positive airway pressure (CPAP) can be used to reduce the workload on the heart and push fluid out of the lungs. For pneumonia, rapid transport to the hospital for antibiotic treatment is vital.

Importance of Rapid Assessment and Action

When dealing with respiratory emergencies, the adage 'time is of the essence' could not be more accurate. Delays in recognizing and addressing respiratory distress can lead to respiratory failure, cardiac arrest, and other life-threatening situations. Consequently, assessing a patient's respiratory status quickly, identifying potential issues, and initiating appropriate treatment is paramount for EMTs. Mastering the knowledge and skills to handle respiratory emergencies is a significant challenge, but it's one that you, as an EMT, are well-equipped to meet. Remember, your actions in these situations can make a substantial difference in your patients' lives, providing them with the vital moments they need to reach definitive care.

Cardiovascular Emergencies

Cardiovascular emergencies represent a significant portion of calls for emergency medical services. Quick, decisive action in these instances can mean the difference between life and death, underlining the importance of a comprehensive understanding of the cardiovascular system and its potential pathologies.

Understanding Cardiovascular Anatomy and Physiology

A robust grasp of the cardiovascular system's structure and function is essential to navigate cardiovascular emergencies effectively. The heart, composed of four chambers, is the core of this intricate system. The heart aims to pump blood throughout the body, supplying cells with oxygen and nutrients while removing waste products. This delicate balance can be disturbed by various conditions, each requiring a unique response.

Identifying Cardiovascular Distress

Recognizing the signs of cardiovascular distress is the first critical step in managing cardiovascular emergencies. The symptoms can be as apparent as chest pain or as subtle as fatigue, dizziness, or nausea. Other vital signs include palpitations, shortness of breath, pain radiating to the left arm or jaw, sweating, and altered mental status. Changes in skin color or temperature and abnormal heart rhythms can also be red flags.

Types of Cardiovascular Emergencies

Understanding the range of potential cardiovascular emergencies is vital. Heart attacks, or myocardial infarctions, occur when a part of the heart muscle is starved of oxygen, often due to a blocked coronary artery. Symptoms may include severe chest pain, shortness of breath, and sweating. Immediate action, including rapid transport to a hospital, is paramount.

Angina, similar to a heart attack, involves chest pain or discomfort due to reduced blood flow to the heart muscle but does not result in permanent heart damage. Cardiac arrhythmias and abnormal heart rhythms may present with palpitations, chest pain, shortness of breath, or fainting. Heart failure, which happens when the heart can't pump enough blood to meet the body's needs, may lead to shortness of breath, fatigue, and swelling of the legs and ankles.

Initial Management and Interventions

The primary initial steps in managing cardiovascular emergencies are similar to those in respiratory distress: ensuring an open airway, assessing vital signs, and providing supplemental oxygen if necessary. Specific interventions may be appropriate for some conditions, such as aspirin administration for suspected myocardial infarction or nitroglycerin for angina. Cardiopulmonary resuscitation (CPR) and an automated external defibrillator (AED) may be required in cases of cardiac arrest.

The Importance of Pre-hospital Care

Time is of the essence in cardiovascular emergencies. The sooner a patient receives appropriate treatment, the better their chances of survival and recovery. As an EMT, you are critical in recognizing these emergencies, initiating lifesaving interventions, and rapidly transporting the patient to the hospital. Each decision you make can impact the outcome, underscoring the significance of your role.

Understanding cardiovascular emergencies may feel overwhelming due to the high stakes and complex medical knowledge involved. However, your training and continual learning equip you to make a tangible difference in these situations. In cardiovascular emergencies, an EMT's skills and knowledge can be life-altering, if not lifesaving, which is a profound testament to the profession's importance.

Diabetic Emergencies

In medical emergencies, diabetic emergencies pose a unique set of challenges. Diabetes, a chronic condition characterized by elevated blood glucose levels, affects millions worldwide and is often a precipitating factor in various acute medical emergencies. As an EMT, understanding the complexities of diabetes and how to address diabetic emergencies is crucial.

Understanding Diabetes

Diabetes is a condition in which the body cannot regulate blood sugar levels properly. This is due to the body's inability to produce insulin (Type 1 diabetes), or it cannot effectively use its insulin (Type 2 diabetes). Insulin is a hormone that allows cells to absorb glucose from the bloodstream and use it for energy. When insulin production or utilization is impaired, blood glucose levels rise, leading to diabetes.

Recognizing Diabetic Emergencies

Diabetic emergencies typically result from extremely high or low blood glucose levels: hyperglycemia and hypoglycemia. Hyperglycemia, high blood glucose, often develops slowly over days or weeks. The patient may present with symptoms like frequent urination, excessive thirst, nausea, vomiting, fatigue, and blurred vision. If untreated, severe hyperglycemia can lead to diabetic ketoacidosis (DKA), a life-threatening condition characterized by high blood sugar, ketone buildup, and acidosis.

Hypoglycemia, low blood glucose, generally develops quickly, often within minutes or hours. It may occur due to excessive insulin, skipped meals, or extra physical activity. Symptoms may include confusion, dizziness, weakness, rapid heart rate, sweating, and unconsciousness. Severe hypoglycemia can lead to seizures or coma.

Initial Management of Diabetic Emergencies

Initial management of diabetic emergencies starts with a primary assessment. If the patient is conscious and able to swallow, offering a sugar source, like fruit juice or glucose gel, can help address hypoglycemia. However, never attempt to give oral glucose to an unconscious patient due to the risk of aspiration.
For hyperglycemic emergencies, initial management primarily focuses on supportive care while arranging for rapid transport to the hospital. It is crucial to remember that you cannot administer insulin in the pre-hospital setting as an EMT.

Documentation and Communication

Diabetic emergencies require detailed documentation and effective communication with incoming hospital staff. Documenting the patient's initial glucose level, any changes in their condition, interventions provided, and their response to those interventions can aid the hospital team in further treating the patient.

The Role of EMTs in Diabetic Emergencies

As an EMT, you play a pivotal role in managing diabetic emergencies. Your actions on the scene can drastically alter the patient's outcome. Quick recognition of the signs and symptoms of hypo and hyperglycemia and timely intervention can mitigate the risk of severe complications. Your ongoing education about diabetes, its manifestations, and its emergencies equips you to provide your patients with the highest level of care. In conclusion, diabetic emergencies constitute a significant percentage of medical calls. Understanding the pathophysiology of diabetes, recognizing the signs and symptoms of diabetic emergencies, and knowing how to manage these conditions in the pre-hospital setting are all essential skills for any EMT preparing for the EMT exam. Despite the high stakes, your comprehensive training and understanding of diabetic emergencies can make a world of difference to your patients, their families, and the community you serve.

Allergic Reactions

One of the most common medical emergencies encountered by emergency medical technicians (EMTs) is allergic reactions, also known as hypersensitivity reactions. Understanding the biological mechanisms, recognizing symptoms, and administering appropriate interventions are essential for an EMT navigating the complexity of these emergencies.

Allergic Reactions

An allergic reaction occurs when the body's immune system overreacts to a foreign substance known as an allergen. Common allergens include foods, medications, insect venom, and environmental factors like pollen or dust mites. Allergic reactions range in severity from mild symptoms, like a runny nose or itchy eyes, to life-threatening conditions, such as anaphylaxis.

Understanding Anaphylaxis

Anaphylaxis is a severe, potentially fatal systemic allergic reaction that can occur within seconds or minutes of exposure to an allergen. It represents a true emergency requiring immediate intervention. Symptoms can affect multiple body systems, including hives, facial or throat swelling, difficulty breathing, rapid pulse, dizziness, or unconsciousness.

Recognizing Allergic Reactions

Prompt recognition of allergic reactions is critical to delivering effective pre-hospital care. Mild allergic reactions may present with localized symptoms such as hives, itchiness, or swelling. However, as the severity of the allergic reaction increases, symptoms become more systemic and can impact the respiratory and cardiovascular systems, leading to difficulty breathing chest tightness, and changes in heart rate and blood pressure.

Initial Management of Allergic Reactions

Initial management of allergic reactions begins with ensuring the scene's safety, conducting a thorough primary assessment, and calling for additional resources if necessary. Mild reactions may only require monitoring and transport to the hospital for further review. However, severe reactions like anaphylaxis demand immediate intervention.

If permitted by your local protocols, administering epinephrine, commonly known as an EpiPen, is the first-line treatment for anaphylaxis. Epinephrine works by narrowing blood vessels and opening airways in the lungs, which can help restore blood pressure, facilitate breathing, decrease hives, and reduce swelling. Remember, the patient's airway, breathing, and circulation should be continually reassessed. Administer high-flow oxygen as required and consider positioning the patient in a way that supports their breathing, such as a semi-Fowler's position.

The Role of EMTs in Allergic Reactions

As an EMT, your actions during an allergic reaction can significantly impact the patient's outcome. Fast identification of symptoms, swift decision-making regarding treatment, and continuous monitoring of the patient's status are all crucial aspects of effective pre-hospital care for allergic reactions.

In conclusion, allergic reactions can evolve rapidly and unpredictably, making them a common and significant concern in emergency medicine. As an EMT, your knowledge about these reactions, from understanding the underlying pathophysiology to delivering timely interventions, can make the difference between life and death. By mastering this content, you can excel in your EMT exam and improve patient outcomes in real-world scenarios. The more prepared you are to tackle these emergencies, the more valuable you become as a healthcare provider, poised to serve your community professionally and skillfully.

Poisoning/Overdose

An important area of focus for emergency medical technicians (EMTs) is recognizing and managing poisoning and overdose emergencies. These situations present unique challenges and can quickly become life-threatening, necessitating a comprehensive understanding of the topic to deliver effective pre-hospital care.

Understanding Poisoning

Poisoning occurs when a harmful substance is ingested, inhaled, injected, or absorbed through the skin, causing harm to the body. Sources of poisons can be numerous, from household chemicals and carbon monoxide to plants, alcohol, and drugs. The severity of poisoning hinges on multiple factors, including the type and quantity of poison, the route of exposure, and the patient's age and health status.

Comprehending Overdose

Overdose, often considered a form of poisoning, occurs when an individual consumes an excessive substance, typically a drug, leading to a harmful physiological response. Overdoses can be intentional, as in suicide attempts or misuse of drugs, or unintentional, such as when a child ingests a medication they mistake for candy.

Recognizing Poisoning and Overdose

Recognizing the signs and symptoms of poisoning or overdose is crucial. While symptoms can vary based on the substance involved, common manifestations include altered mental status, seizures, difficulty breathing, chest or abdominal pain, nausea, vomiting, and changes in pupil size. Signs of specific toxic syndromes (toxidromes), like pinpoint pupils in opioid overdose or dilated pupils in stimulant use, can aid identification of the offending substance.

Initial Management of Poisoning/Overdose

The initial response to poisoning or overdose starts with scene safety. Some substances pose risks to rescuers, so ensuring proper protective measures is paramount. Next, perform a rapid primary assessment, focusing on the airway, breathing, and circulation. Depending on local protocols, administer oxygen and consider using antidotes if the substance is known and treatment is available.

Some poisoning cases might require activated charcoal, which binds to the poison in the stomach to limit absorption into the body. However, its use is not universal and should be directed by medical directions or local protocols.

For overdose cases, particularly opioid overdoses, naloxone (Narcan) can reverse the effects of opioids and restore normal respiration. Nevertheless, it should be used judiciously, considering its potential to precipitate withdrawal symptoms in chronic opioid users.

Patient Assessment and Transport

A thorough history and physical exam can reveal vital information about the substance and exposure timeline. Bring samples of the substance or its container to the hospital if possible. Immediate transport is essential for all but the most minor cases of poisoning or overdose.

EMTs' Role in Poisoning/Overdose

As an EMT, your primary roles in poisoning and overdose cases are to recognize the situation, initiate appropriate care, and rapidly transport the patient to the hospital. Timely interventions can be lifesaving, especially in severe systemic poisoning or overdose cases.

Conclusively, poisoning and overdose emergencies can be complex, requiring EMTs to apply their knowledge of toxicology, patient assessment, and emergency care. Being prepared to respond effectively to these emergencies not only aids in passing the EMT exam but also contributes to improved patient outcomes. Remember, your actions as an EMT can make a significant difference in the health and survival of a patient dealing with poisoning or overdose.

SPECIAL POPULATIONS

Regarding emergency medical care, it's critical to recognize that each patient is unique. However, some groups require distinct considerations based on age, medical conditions, or other factors. We refer to these groups as "special populations." These include pediatric and geriatric patients, patients with special healthcare needs, and pregnant patients. As an Emergency Medical Technician (EMT), understanding how to approach and manage the needs of these special populations is fundamental.

Pediatric Patients

Pediatric patients are not just small adults. Their physiological responses to illness and injury can be vastly different. Children's airways are narrower, and their metabolic rates are higher. They can compensate for shock longer, but their condition can rapidly deteriorate once they decompensate. In addition to these physical differences, it's crucial to communicate effectively with children to reduce fear and gain cooperation.

Treatment strategies should be age-appropriate, considering the child's developmental and cognitive level. For example, engaging with a toddler differently than with a school-aged child might be necessary. Rapid, safe transport to a pediatric-capable facility is crucial for severe illness or injury.

Geriatric Patients

As people age, their bodies undergo numerous changes that can impact their response to illness and injury. Geriatric patients often have multiple chronic conditions, take several medications, and may have sensory or cognitive impairments. These factors can make assessment and management more complex. For example, a geriatric patient with a minor head injury might be at higher risk for complications due to blood-thinning medication. In caring for geriatric patients, remember that they might need more time to understand and respond. Be patient and respectful, and always consider the possibility of elder abuse or neglect in unexplained injuries or poor living conditions.

Patients with Special Healthcare Needs

Patients with special healthcare needs may have physical, developmental, or cognitive disabilities that require tailored approaches in emergency care. This can include patients with tracheostomies, feeding tubes, or those who use a wheelchair. Understanding the function and care needs of their specialized medical equipment is crucial. Communication can also be challenging, requiring patience and creative solutions.

Pregnant Patients

Pregnant patients present unique challenges in emergency care. Changes in anatomy and physiology during pregnancy can affect the patient's response to treatment. For instance, a pregnant patient might need to be positioned on her left side to prevent compression of the vena cava, which can lead to decreased blood flow to the heart and potential loss of consciousness.

Emergencies can involve the mother, the unborn child, or both, ranging from minor injuries to severe complications like eclampsia or placental abruption. Quick identification of the pregnancy and the potential related complications is crucial.

Culturally Diverse Patients

Effective emergency care includes respecting cultural differences and beliefs. EMTs must know about cultural sensitivities, language barriers, and traditional practices. When possible, use interpreter services or family members to bridge language gaps. Also, be aware of cultural practices that might impact patient care, such as preferences about the gender of the healthcare provider.

End of Life Patients

Patients at the end of life or terminal illnesses also require special considerations. They may have advanced directives or do-not-resuscitate orders. EMTs should be familiar with local laws and protocols regarding these orders. Furthermore, showing empathy and understanding can go a long way in comforting these patients and their loved ones.

In conclusion, effectively caring for special populations is a vital skill for EMTs. Each patient's unique circumstances require thoughtful, individualized care. By recognizing and understanding these differences, you can ensure that your treatment aligns with each patient's needs, upholding the standards of compassionate and professional emergency medical care.

Obstetrics and Neonatal Care

Obstetrics and neonatal care hold an essential place in emergency medical services. As an Emergency Medical Technician (EMT), you often attend to pregnancy-related emergencies and neonatal care situations. These scenarios require specialized knowledge and skills to ensure the well-being of both the mother and the infant.

Understanding Obstetric Emergencies

Obstetric emergencies refer to life-threatening complications arising during pregnancy, childbirth, or postpartum. These include preterm labor, placental abruption, preeclampsia, and postpartum hemorrhage. In these emergencies, your priority is stabilizing the mother while arranging immediate hospital transport. Proper management of obstetric emergencies often depends on early recognition of the signs and symptoms, accurate assessment of the mother and fetus, and prompt initiation of treatment protocols.

Preterm Labor and Delivery

Preterm labor, occurring before 37 weeks of gestation, can lead to premature birth, presenting risks to the infant, like respiratory distress syndrome, neonatal sepsis, and neurological complications. Warning signs include regular contractions, rupture of membranes (known colloquially as the 'water breaking'), and pelvic pressure. If delivery appears imminent, prepare for a field delivery while expediting transport.

Placental Abruption and Placenta Previa

Both placental abruption, where the placenta detaches from the uterus prematurely, and placenta previa, where the placenta lies unusually low in the uterus, can cause severe maternal hemorrhage. These conditions present with vaginal bleeding, with placental abruption often associated with severe abdominal pain. Both necessitate rapid transport, as they can pose an immediate danger to the mother and baby.

Preeclampsia and Eclampsia

Preeclampsia is a pregnancy-specific syndrome of hypertension and organ dysfunction, and eclampsia includes the onset of seizures in a patient with preeclampsia. Symptoms may include severe headaches, visual disturbances, high blood pressure, and upper abdominal pain. Eclampsia is a life-threatening condition that warrants immediate transport and hospital management.

Postpartum Hemorrhage

Postpartum hemorrhage is excessive bleeding following delivery, often resulting from the uterus failing to contract properly after childbirth. It is a significant cause of maternal mortality worldwide and requires immediate treatment.

Neonatal Care

Care for newborns, particularly those born preterm or with complications, presents unique challenges. Neonatal resuscitation might be required if the baby does not breathe or has a heart rate of less than 100 beats per minute after birth.

Understanding the neonatal resuscitation protocol, including providing warmth, positioning the airway, clearing the airway if needed, drying, stimulating, and reassessing, is critical. Neonates lose heat quickly, and hypothermia can exacerbate existing problems. Thus, keeping the newborn warm is essential.

Remember, neonates often require gentler, more precise interventions. For example, when providing ventilations, use a neonate-sized bag-valve-mask device, give smaller breaths, and ventilate faster than adults.

Providing care in obstetric emergencies and neonatal situations requires specific knowledge, a calm demeanor, and decisive action. Swift recognition of conditions, immediate initiation of care, and rapid transport to an appropriate medical facility can significantly impact outcomes. Although the situations may be high-pressure, the opportunity to bring new life safely into the world or to protect that life in its earliest stages is one of the most rewarding aspects of the EMT's role.

Pediatric Emergencies

Pediatric emergencies present unique challenges for Emergency Medical Technicians (EMTs). Kids are not simply miniature adults; they have distinct physiological differences and often communicate their needs differently. The severity of their condition can change rapidly, making them a particularly vulnerable population. Recognizing these differences and understanding how to approach pediatric patients is crucial in an emergency.

Physiological Differences in Pediatric Patients

Understanding the physiological differences between children and adults is crucial in a pediatric emergency. These differences affect everything from the etiology of their conditions to the way they respond to treatment.

Children have higher metabolic rates and can become hypoxic faster than adults. Their airways are narrower and can become obstructed more easily. Their body surface area is larger relative to their weight, making them more prone to hypothermia. And their circulatory system responds differently to shock, often compensating longer but then decompensating rapidly.

Assessment and Management

Remember the importance of a gentle, calm approach when assessing a pediatric patient. Many children are frightened in emergencies and may not understand what's happening. Be mindful of your body language and tone of voice.

Start with a hands-off approach, observing the child's appearance, work of breathing, and circulation to the skin. The pediatric assessment follows the same ABCDE structure as adults, but remember to use age-appropriate norms for vital signs.

Remember that children can compensate during shock and may appear stable until they reach a critical point. Recognizing the early signs of pediatric shock, such as altered mental status, tachycardia, and delayed capillary refill, can be lifesaving.

Common Pediatric Emergencies

There are various pediatric emergencies that an EMT may encounter. Respiratory distress is expected due to asthma, croup, or foreign body aspiration. As respiratory distress can quickly lead to respiratory failure in children, prompt identification and treatment are vital.

Febrile seizures, associated with rapid temperature increases, are another typical emergency in the pediatric population. Although generally benign, they can be frightening to witness, and the EMT's role includes reassuring the caregivers while ensuring the child's safety during the seizure.

Additionally, children are prone to certain types of injuries due to their size, level of development, and curiosity. These include burns, falls, and ingestions of harmful substances.

Pediatric emergencies can be among the most challenging calls an EMT responds to, mainly due to the unique physiological and psychological aspects of treating children. A solid understanding of these differences and the ability to quickly assess and treat pediatric patients can significantly improve the outcome of these emergencies.

Finally, always appreciate the importance of emotional support and reassurance for the child and their caregivers. They are an integral part of the process and can play a significant role in the child's recovery.

Geriatric Patients

As our population ages, emergency medical services (EMS) increasingly encounter geriatric patients aged 65 and over. Caring for this population presents unique challenges due to their complex medical histories, multiple medications, and varied physiological responses to injury and illness. As an Emergency Medical Technician (EMT), understanding the unique considerations of geriatric patients is essential to provide the most effective care.

Recognizing the Unique Physiology of Geriatric Patients

Geriatric patients differ physiologically from younger adults. As we age, all body systems gradually decline in function. These changes can complicate the response to emergencies and the management of chronic conditions.

For instance, older adults typically have decreased lung elasticity and weakened muscles of respiration, which can exacerbate conditions like pneumonia or Chronic Obstructive Pulmonary Disease (COPD). Their hearts may not respond as effectively to stress, putting them at risk during acute events. The kidneys' ability to filter and excrete waste diminishes, impacting medication dosages and the risk of toxicity.

Moreover, the neurological changes associated with aging can mask the signs and symptoms of severe conditions. For instance, elderly patients may not exhibit the typical signs of a heart attack. Instead of chest pain, they may feel generalized weakness, fatigue, or confusion, making the diagnosis more challenging.

The Complex Medical History and Polypharmacy

Older adults often have a complicated medical history with multiple co-existing chronic diseases. It's common for geriatric patients to manage conditions like hypertension, diabetes, heart disease, arthritis, and cognitive disorders concurrently.

Further complicating the picture is polypharmacy – the use of multiple medications to manage these chronic conditions. Keeping track of these medications, understanding their interactions, and recognizing their potential side effects are crucial to the EMT's assessment.

Assessment and Management of Geriatric Patients

When assessing geriatric patients, consider their overall health status and baseline function. It's important to remember that 'normal' vital signs may differ in this population – for instance, slightly elevated blood pressure might be expected for an older patient.

Obtaining a thorough patient history is critical. Pay special attention to any changes in mental status, which can often indicate a severe underlying problem in geriatric patients. Also, consider potential trauma from falls, common in older people due to balance issues and decreased bone density.

Communication is critical. Many older patients may have hearing or vision impairments, so speak clearly and ensure they understand the situation and your actions. Where possible, involve family members or caregivers who can provide valuable insight into the patient's normal behavior and health status.

Geriatric-Specific Emergencies

Specific emergencies are more common in geriatric patients. Falls are a significant concern, often resulting from balance issues, muscle weakness, or medication side effects. Even minor falls can lead to severe injuries like hip fractures or traumatic brain injuries due to the fragility of the elderly.

Elderly patients are also more prone to pneumonia and urinary tract infections. Importantly, these can often present without the typical symptoms – an older person with a urinary tract infection may not complain of pain or frequency but instead appear confused.

Caring for geriatric patients requires a keen understanding of the physiological changes of aging, a thorough and patient approach to assessment, and excellent communication skills. As an EMT, you'll play a crucial role in recognizing and managing emergencies in this vulnerable population, making a real difference in their health outcomes. Always treat your geriatric patients with the same respect and dignity you would want for your loved ones. These skills will only become more vital as we continue to serve an aging population.

EMS OPERATIONS

I n Emergency Medical Services (EMS), successful patient outcomes depend not only on the clinical expertise of the EMTs but also on effective EMS operations. These operations encompass everything from when a call comes into the dispatch center, through the on-scene care and transport of a patient, to the handover at the receiving hospital. Understanding the intricacies of EMS operations is essential for any EMT preparing for their exam and career.

EMS System Overview

The EMS system is a complex, coordinated response and medical care network involving multiple agencies and individuals. At its heart is the goal of providing emergency medical care to those in need, whether due to sudden illness, injury, or disaster.

Dispatchers triage the situation upon receiving a call for help, determining the appropriate response level and resources needed. Trained EMTs then respond, providing initial care, stabilization, and transport while coordinating with hospital staff to ensure a seamless transition of care.

Communications and Dispatch

The efficiency of EMS operations hinges significantly on effective communication. This communication begins with the dispatch center, the primary hub for emergency call intake, triage, and resource deployment.

Dispatchers use established protocols to categorize calls according to their severity, determining the required EMS response level. They also provide pre-arrival instructions to callers, guiding them to perform crucial interventions such as CPR.

EMTs must maintain open lines of communication with dispatchers, responding to updates about the situation and informing the dispatcher of their status.

Scene Size-Up and Safety

Upon arrival, the EMT's priority is to 'size up' the scene, assessing the situation for safety and understanding what might have caused the patient's condition. Scene safety is paramount; an unsafe location can pose risks to EMTs, patients, and bystanders.

Possible dangers include traffic, fire, hazardous materials, violence, or unstable structures. If a scene is unsafe, EMTs must wait for it to be secured before proceeding, communicating with other responding agencies as needed.

Patient Assessment and Care

Practical patient assessment and care lie at the heart of EMS operations. EMTs must quickly assess the patient's condition, identify life-threatening issues, and initiate appropriate interventions.
The patient assessment process includes the primary survey (ABCs – Airway, Breathing, Circulation), history taking, and the secondary survey, a head-to-toe examination to identify injuries or conditions that may not be immediately life-threatening but still require treatment. EMTs provide treatment according to their scope of practice and protocols, intending to stabilize the patient for transport.

Coordination with Other Agencies

EMS often works with other agencies, such as fire departments, police, and specialty response teams. Effective coordination with these agencies is essential to ensure scene safety, patient care, and the efficient use of resources.

Transport and Transfer of Care

After providing initial care, EMTs prepare the patient for transport. During transport, EMTs monitor the patient, reassess their condition, and provide ongoing maintenance. Upon arrival at the hospital, EMTs must effectively transfer care to the hospital staff. This process includes providing verbal and written patient care reports, ensuring that the hospital team understands the patient's condition, the care provided, and any changes during transport.

Quality Improvement

Quality improvement is a continuous process in EMS, aiming to enhance patient care. It involves reviewing patient care reports, analyzing performance, and identifying areas where the service can improve. EMS operations are a critical aspect of providing high-quality emergency care. It's not just about knowing how to perform medical procedures; it's about understanding the entire operational process, from dispatch to transport and everything in between. This knowledge ensures that EMTs can provide the most efficient and effective care possible, ultimately improving patient outcomes.

Ambulance Operations

A critical aspect of EMS operations is the operation of the ambulance itself. Efficient ambulance operations can dramatically impact patient outcomes. Knowing how to handle ambulance operations appropriately can mean the difference between life and death for an EMT.

Ambulance and Equipment Familiarity

Before operating an ambulance, an EMT should familiarize themselves with the vehicle and its equipment. Different ambulances have different layouts and systems, and understanding where everything is located and how to operate it can save critical time in an emergency. This includes understanding the ambulance's medical equipment, such as the oxygen system, suction devices, monitors, and automated external defibrillators (AEDs).

Emergency Vehicle Operations

Driving an ambulance is different from driving a regular vehicle. It's larger, heavier, and you'll often drive at high speeds in challenging conditions. EMTs must be familiar with how their particular ambulance handles and the driving techniques required to navigate traffic and adverse weather safely. This includes understanding the principles of defensive driving and using lights and sirens appropriately. Misuse of lights and sirens can lead to accidents and delayed patient care, so EMTs should follow their local protocols regarding their use.

Scene Approach and Positioning

How an ambulance is positioned at a scene can impact safety and patient care. The ambulance should be set to protect the scene, especially on busy roadways, without blocking other responding units. An EMT should consider potential hazards and ensure the ambulance is not placed in a dangerous position.

Patient Loading and Unloading

Proper patient loading and unloading procedures are vital for patient safety. Patients should be secured in the ambulance to prevent injury during transport, and EMTs should use proper lifting techniques to avoid back damage.

EMTs should also consider the patient's condition when determining the best method for loading and unloading. For example, a patient with a suspected spinal injury must be loaded onto a long spine board before being moved into the ambulance.

On-Scene Operations

While on the scene, EMTs must coordinate with other responders, communicate with dispatch, perform patient assessments and interventions, and prepare the patient for transport. This requires multi-tasking and situational awareness to complete all tasks efficiently and effectively.

Transport Considerations

During transport, EMTs must continue to care for the patient, monitor their condition, and communicate with the receiving facility. Transport speed should be determined based on the patient's condition, and EMTs should consider potential traffic and road conditions when deciding on the best route to the hospital.

Transfer of Care

Once at the hospital, the EMT must effectively transfer care to the hospital staff. This involves giving a verbal report about the patient's condition, the care provided, and any changes during transport. The EMT will also need to complete a written patient care report detailing all patient care aspects.

Post-Transport Responsibilities

After transport, EMTs have several responsibilities. They must restock the ambulance and clean any equipment used. They should also disinfect the patient compartment if they have a communicable disease. Additionally, EMTs should participate in debriefings or critical incident stress management sessions as necessary.

Ambulance Safety

Safety is a paramount concern in ambulance operations. This includes wearing seat belts when the vehicle is in motion, using appropriate personal protective equipment, and adhering to safe driving practices.

Operating an ambulance requires more than just driving skills. It's a multifaceted process that involves scene management, patient care, communication, and logistics. It's about navigating the dynamic emergency care environment while safely and quickly getting patients the needed help. As an EMT, mastering these aspects of ambulance operations is crucial to providing the best possible care to your patients.

Gaining Access and Patient Extrication

A critical part of EMS operations involves gaining access to patients and, when necessary, extricating them from confined or hazardous situations. Often, the physical location or circumstances of a medical emergency require EMTs to deploy specific strategies and use specialized equipment to reach and safely remove patients.

Understanding the Need for Access and Extrication

EMTs may be called to various scenes, such as vehicle collisions, industrial accidents, or situations involving falls from heights. The challenge here is to provide medical care and gain access to the patient safely and efficiently. In some instances, patients may need to be extricated – that is, removed from a hazardous situation or location or inhibits effective treatment.

Scene Safety and Size-up

The first step in any access or extrication operation is to ensure the safety of everyone present, including the patient, bystanders, and emergency personnel. This begins with a scene size-up, an initial evaluation to identify potential hazards, the number and condition of patients, and the resources required.

Gaining Access

Once the scene is deemed safe, EMTs gain access to the patient. This might involve using hand tools, such as a window punch or seat belt cutter in vehicle extrication, or more complex equipment like hydraulic rescue tools (commonly known as the Jaws of Life) when doors or other barriers cannot be quickly or safely opened. During this phase, EMTS must use appropriate personal protective equipment (PPE), including gloves, helmets, and eye protection.

Patient Assessment and Care

Once access is gained, EMTs must quickly assess the patient's condition. Vital signs are monitored, and primary and secondary surveys are performed to identify injuries. EMTS must stabilize any life-threatening conditions, provide initial treatment, and prepare the patient for extrication.

Patient Extrication

Extrication involves the safe removal of the patient from the entrapment. Depending on the situation's complexity, it might require the coordinated efforts of several responders. During extrication, care is taken to prevent further injury, especially to the spine. Thus, immobilization devices like cervical collars, backboards, and scoop stretchers may be used. The chosen method often depends on the patient's condition, the degree of entrapment, and the available resources.

Post-Extrication Care

After extrication, the patient is reassessed, and care continues during transport. This is the time to address any injuries or conditions that were not immediately life-threatening but now require attention. A detailed physical exam is conducted, and the patient's vital signs are closely monitored.

Coordinating with Other Agencies

Access and extrication operations often involve coordination with other agencies, such as fire departments or specialized rescue teams. Inter-agency communication and cooperation are essential for successful operations. EMTs need to understand their role in the more extensive process and how to interact with other agencies effectively.

Documentation

Like all EMS operations, gaining access and patient extrication must be thoroughly documented. The patient care report (PCR) should include details of the incident, including how access was achieved, the method of extrication, the patient's initial condition, treatment given, and any changes in condition.

Training and Education

Access and extrication techniques often require specialized training and ongoing education. EMTs must keep updated on the latest procedures, equipment, and guidelines, reinforcing their knowledge with practical, hands-on training. Gaining access and patient extrication is a complex yet crucial aspect of EMS operations. It requires a comprehensive set of skills, ranging from scene assessment and safety protocols to patient care and inter-agency cooperation. Above all, EMTs must always commit to their primary goal – the safe and efficient delivery of patients to definitive care. As an EMT, understanding and applying these principles will prepare you for challenging yet rewarding situations.

Hazardous Materials Incidents

When hazardous materials are involved in incidents, it calls for a particular response from EMTs. Due to the potential for severe harm or environmental damage, these situations require a unique set of knowledge, skills, and procedures. Let's explore how EMTs respond to these challenging scenarios.

Recognizing Hazardous Materials Incidents

The first step in managing a hazardous materials incident is recognition. EMTs might be called to a known dangerous materials incident, such as a chemical plant explosion or a transportation accident involving marked containers. But it's also crucial to be vigilant for signs of hazardous materials in less obvious situations. Clues might include unusual odors, unexplained physical symptoms in patients or bystanders, or materials that look out of place.

Safety First: The Concept of Time, Distance, and Shielding

Once a hazardous materials incident is recognized, the safety of the EMT, the patient, and any bystanders is prioritized. The concept of time, distance, and shielding is applied. Minimize the time spent in the hazardous area, maximize the distance from the source of the hazard, and use appropriate shielding or barriers to protect against exposure.

Calling for Specialized Resources

Hazardous materials incidents often exceed the training and capabilities of EMTs. When faced with such an incident, calling for assistance from specialized dangerous materials response teams is crucial. These teams have the training and equipment to manage the incident and provide advanced care if needed safely.

Initial Isolation and Protective Actions

While waiting for specialized resources, there are steps that EMTs can take to improve safety. Establishing an initial isolation zone prevents uncontrolled access to the hazardous area. Protective actions include evacuating nearby bystanders or instructing them to take shelter.

Identifying the Material

Knowing the type of material involved in the incident can help EMTs and other responders make better decisions. The Department of Transportation's Emergency Response Guidebook (ERG) is valuable. The ERG provides critical information about the hazards, recommended protective actions, and first aid measures by cross-referencing placards, container shapes, or other identifiers.

Decontamination and Patient Care

Decontamination, or removing hazardous substances from people and equipment, may be necessary before patient care can proceed. Decontamination procedures vary based on the material and exposure but often involve removing contaminated clothing and flushing exposed skin and eyes with water.

The same principles of ABC (Airway, Breathing, Circulation) apply to patient care. However, treatments might be modified based on the material involved and the potential for secondary contamination of personnel or equipment. The ERG and online resources like the Toxicological Profiles from the Agency for Toxic Substances and Disease Registry can provide specific guidance.

Reporting and Documentation

As with any EMS operation, proper reporting and documentation are critical. A detailed patient care report (PCR) helps ensure continuity of care, facilitates further investigation, and provides a record for legal and administrative purposes. In addition to the standard elements of a PCR, the report should include details of the hazardous material, decontamination measures, and any changes in the patient's condition.

Training and Education

Hazardous materials incidents require specialized training. EMTs should understand their local protocols and have regular education and drills. At a minimum, EMTs need training at the Operations level, which includes recognizing hazardous materials incidents, initiating protective actions, and calling for appropriate resources.

Hazardous materials incidents are a unique challenge in EMS operations. While these incidents are rare, EMTs must be prepared to respond safely and effectively. EMTs play a critical role in managing these complex incidents by recognizing the potential for hazardous materials, taking appropriate protective actions, coordinating with specialized resources, and providing patient care within their scope of practice.

Multiple-Casualty Incidents

Multiple-casualty incidents (MCIs) are situations where the number and severity of patients outstrip the immediately available resources. While rare for an EMT, these events pose distinct challenges requiring exceptional preparedness, efficient resource management, and triage skills.

Understanding Multiple-Casualty Incidents

MCIs can arise from various situations, ranging from traffic accidents and structural collapses to mass shootings and natural disasters. Each of these situations presents unique problems, but they all share the common issue of needing to deliver effective care to many patients simultaneously.

Planning for MCIs

MCIs require a different approach compared to routine EMS operations. To manage these incidents, EMTs should be well-versed in incident management concepts, such as the Incident Command System (ICS). ICS provides a standardized, on-scene, all-hazards approach to incident management, enabling coordination and cooperation among agencies and responders.

Activation of MCI Protocol

When an MCI is identified, EMTs or other first responders will activate the MCI protocol. This action triggers a series of steps to ensure that resources are mobilized appropriately, including notifying hospitals, activating additional EMS resources, and possibly declaring a state of emergency.

Triage in MCIs

The core of managing an MCI is triage. Triage, derived from the French word "trier," meaning "to sort," is a process of quickly assessing each patient's condition and assigning a priority level. The goal is to do the greatest good for the most significant number of patients, sometimes providing minimal care or delaying care for some patients to save others. The most common triage system in the U.S. is Simple Triage and Rapid Treatment (START). Using the START system, patients are categorized as red (immediate), yellow (delayed), green (minor), or black (deceased/expectant) based on their ability to walk, respiratory status, perfusion, and mental status.

Patient Management and Transport

Once triaged, patients are moved to treatment areas based on their priority level. Emergency medical care is then provided according to established protocols and resource availability. The aim is to stabilize patients and prepare them for transport. Regarding transportation, priority goes to the most critical patients who can survive. In coordination with hospitals and transportation resources, the Incident Commander directs patient transport to avoid overwhelming any single hospital.

Communication

During an MCI, effective communication is crucial. This involves not just communication among responders at the scene but also with hospitals, dispatch centers, and potentially the media and the public. Incident Commanders and Public Information Officers (PIOs) typically handle most of this communication.

Documenting and Debriefing

As in any EMS operation, proper documentation is critical in an MCI. In addition to individual patient care reports, responders may be asked to contribute to an incident report detailing their actions and observations. After the incident, debriefing sessions and after-action reports help to review the response, identify strengths and weaknesses, and make improvements for future incidents.

MCIs represent one of the most significant challenges in EMS operations. They require EMTs to apply their skills and knowledge in an environment of heightened complexity and pressure. By understanding the principles of MCIs and practicing these skills regularly, EMTs can be better prepared to respond when these events occur, ultimately saving more lives.

EMS Response to Terrorism

In today's world, the threat of terrorism is an unfortunate reality. For an emergency medical technician (EMT), understanding the role of EMS in responding to such incidents is crucial. Whether it's a mass shooting, bombing, or chemical attack, the principles of EMS response to terrorism focus on ensuring personal safety, scene security, and patient care.

Recognizing and Responding to Terrorism Incidents

When arriving at a potential terrorism scene, EMTs must remain vigilant, identifying signs of potential hazards such as unattended items, unusual smells or sounds, or people exhibiting signs of distress. Ensuring personal safety is the primary concern; hence, EMTs must avoid rushing into the scene but adopt a cautious, methodical approach to assessing and managing the incident.

The Stages of Response

There are four primary stages in an EMS response to a terrorism incident:

1. **Preparation**: Preparation is vital and includes familiarization with common types of terrorist attacks and associated hazards, including explosives, firearms, biological and chemical agents, and nuclear materials. EMTs should participate in drills and exercises simulating various types of attacks to enhance their readiness.
2. **Response:** The immediate response to a terrorism incident focuses on ensuring personal safety, scene assessment, resource activation, and patient triage. An emphasis is placed on identifying and addressing immediate life threats while ensuring that the scene is safe for EMS personnel and patients.
3. **Recovery:** During the recovery stage, efforts focus on patient treatment and transport, scene clearance, and initiation of investigative and rescue operations.
4. **Mitigation:** This stage includes actions to prevent future incidents and reduce the impact of those that occur. This could involve reviewing response protocols, providing additional training, or implementing new safety measures.

Incident Command System (ICS) and Terrorism Incidents

The Incident Command System (ICS) is central to managing terrorism incidents. The ICS provides a structured approach to incident management, allowing for effective coordination among multiple agencies and efficient resource utilization.

Patient Care in Terrorism Incidents

Providing patient care during a terrorism incident presents unique challenges. In addition to the physical injuries that can result from explosions or gunfire, psychological trauma may be associated with the event. Furthermore, if the event involves a chemical, biological, radiological, nuclear, or explosive (CBRNE) device, there are additional considerations for patient decontamination and treatment.

Communication in Terrorism Incidents

Effective communication is critical in the management of terrorism incidents. EMTs must be able to communicate with other responders, hospitals, and possibly with law enforcement and other agencies involved in the incident. The information must be shared quickly and accurately to ensure an effective response.

Documentation and Debriefing

Thorough documentation of the EMS response to a terrorism incident is essential for legal, clinical, and operational reasons. After the incident, a debriefing session allows responders to review the incident, identify strengths and weaknesses in the response, and suggest improvements for the future.

Responding to terrorism incidents is a critical aspect of EMS operations. By understanding the fundamental principles and practices associated with these types of incidents, EMTs can help ensure they are prepared to respond effectively, protect themselves and others, and provide appropriate patient care. Though the circumstances are challenging, with adequate preparation and training, EMTs can significantly mitigate the human impact of such events.

PRACTICE TEST

Airway Management

1. Which technique is used to open the airway in an unconscious patient without suspected spinal injury?
   A) Chin-Lift
   B) Jaw-Thrust
   C) Head Tilt-Chin Lift
   D) Tongue-Jaw Lift

2. What does the "C" in ABCs of emergency medicine stand for?
   A) Cardiac
   B) Consciousness
   C) Circulation
   D) Compression

3. What is the primary purpose of the oropharyngeal airway (OPA)?
   A) Ventilation
   B) Oxygenation
   C) Protecting the airway
   D) Suctioning

4. Which of the following is NOT a sign of adequate breathing in an adult?
   A) Regular breath rhythm
   B) Use of accessory muscles
   C) Adequate breath depth
   D) Normal breath sounds

5. Which airway adjunct is contraindicated in conscious patients?
   A) Nasopharyngeal airway (NPA)
   B) Oropharyngeal airway (OPA)
   C) Bag-valve-mask (BVM)
   D) Endotracheal tube (ETT)

6. When suctioning the airway, the suction should not last longer than:
   A) 5 seconds
   B) 10 seconds
   C) 15 seconds
   D) 20 seconds

7. The best position to manage the airway of an unconscious patient without suspected spinal injury is:
   A) Supine
   B) Prone
   C) Recovery Position
   D) Fetal Position

8. Which of the following is NOT an indication of endotracheal intubation?
   A) Need for airway protection
   B) Ineffective ventilation
   C) Need for suctioning
   D) Respiratory arrest

9. What should you do if you hear gurgling while assessing a patient's airway?
   A) Perform chest compressions
   B) Begin ventilations
   C) Suction the airway
   D) Administer oxygen

10. Capnography is used to measure:
    A) Oxygen saturation
    B) Heart rate
    C) End-tidal CO2
    D) Blood pressure

11. When using a bag-valve-mask (BVM), what is the correct ratio of breaths to compressions for a lone rescuer performing CPR on an adult?
    A) 15:2
    B) 5:1
    C) 30:2
    D) 10:1

12. Which patients most likely benefit from using a nasopharyngeal airway (NPA)?
    A) A patient with facial trauma
    B) A conscious patient with a gag reflex
    C) An unconscious patient without a gag reflex
    D) A patient with a known nasal fracture

13. What is the primary purpose of cricoid pressure during endotracheal intubation?
    A) To align the vocal cords
    B) To prevent gastric contents from entering the lungs
    C) To stop bleeding in the throat
    D) To increase oxygen flow

14. What type of airway is generally contraindicated in patients with suspected basal skull fractures?
    A) Oropharyngeal airway (OPA)
    B) Nasopharyngeal airway (NPA)
    C) Endotracheal tube (ETT)
    D) Laryngeal mask airway (LMA)

15. What is the correct placement of the oropharyngeal airway (OPA)?
    A) It extends from the corner of the mouth to the earlobe.
    B) It extends from the tip of the nose to the tragus of the ear.
    C) It extends from the corner of the mouth to the angle of the jaw.
    D) It extends from the tip of the nose to the angle of the jaw.

Patient Assessment

1. The primary survey of a patient begins with which step?
   A) Assessing circulation
   B) Assessing breathing
   C) Assessing the airway
   D) Checking responsiveness

2. What does the acronym SAMPLE stand for in the EMT patient assessment?
   A) Signs, Allergies, Medication, Past medical history, Last oral intake, Events leading up to present illness
   B) Symptoms, Allergies, Medication, Past medical history, Last oral intake, Events leading up to present illness
   C) Signs, Assessment, Medical history, Pulse, Last oral intake, Events leading up to present illness
   D) Symptoms, Assessment, Medication, Pulse, Last oral intake, Events leading up to present illness

3. Which part of the patient assessment focuses on obtaining a detailed history?
   A) Primary Survey
   B) Secondary Survey
   C) Reassessment
   D) Rapid Trauma Assessment

4. Which of the following is NOT a vital sign typically checked by an EMT during a patient assessment?
   A) Blood pressure
   B) Heart rate
   C) Respiratory rate
   D) Blood glucose level

5. What is the primary purpose of the Glasgow Coma Scale (GCS)?
   A) To assess the level of consciousness
   B) To determine the severity of traumatic brain injury
   C) To evaluate a patient's responsiveness to pain
   D) To gauge the extent of a patient's neurological impairment

6. During the primary survey, the rapid trauma assessment is typically conducted on:
   A) All patients
   B) Trauma patients with significant mechanisms of injury
   C) Patients with a history of cardiac arrest
   D) Patients who are unresponsive or have an altered mental status

7. What does OPQRST stand for in patient history taking?
   A) Onset, Provocation, Quality, Region/Radiation, Severity, Time
   B) Onset, Provocation, Quality, Region/Radiation, Signs/Symptoms, Time
   C) Onset, Provocation, Quality, Relief, Severity, Time
   D) Onset, Provocation/Palliation, Quality, Region/Radiation, Severity, Treatment

8. The last vital sign to change in a pediatric patient typically is:
   A) Pulse
   B) Respiration
   C) Blood pressure
   D) Temperature

9. During patient assessment, cyanosis is a sign of:
   A) High blood pressure
   B) Inadequate breathing
   C) Fever
   D) Dehydration

10. In the mnemonic PASTE used for assessing patients with breathing difficulties, what does "E" represent?
    A) Exertion
    B) Exercise
    C) Evaluation
    D) Exacerbation

11. A detailed physical exam should be conducted:
    A) Only if a rapid physical exam has been done
    B) Only on responsive patients
    C) Only on unresponsive patients
    D) Regardless of the patient's mental status

12. The "TIC" in PITCO stands for:
    A) Tenderness, Instability, Crepitus
    B) Trauma, Inflammation, Congestion
    C) Tissue, Integrity, Circulation
    D) Temperature, Intensity, Condition

13. During a patient assessment, which observations should make an EMT suspect a stroke?
    A) Blood pressure is 90/60 mmHg
    B) Pulse is 120 beats per minute
    C) One-sided weakness or facial drooping
    D) Skin is hot and dry

14. During a rapid trauma assessment, an EMT's palpation of the abdomen is primarily for:
    A) Identifying the specific internal organ that may be injured
    B) Checking for the presence of a distended bladder
    C) Detecting any areas of pain, distention, or rigidity
    D) Assessing the patient's level of consciousness

Medical Emergencies

1. In managing a patient with suspected acute myocardial infarction, which should be administered first?
   A) Aspirin
   B) Nitroglycerin
   C) Oxygen
   D) Morphine

2. What is the primary symptom of hypoglycemia?
   A) High blood sugar levels
   B) Uncontrolled hunger
   C) Tremors and weakness
   D) Fruity breath odor

3. An EMT would recognize that a patient is suffering from a syncopal episode by the presence of which of the following?
   A) Chest pain
   B) Sudden loss of consciousness
   C) Increased heart rate
   D) High blood pressure

4. What should an EMT do when encountering a patient showing signs of an allergic reaction first?
   A) Administer an epinephrine auto-injector
   B) Administer antihistamine
   C) Check airway, breathing, and circulation
   D) Apply a cold compress to the affected area

5. Which breath sounds would likely be heard in a patient experiencing a severe asthma attack?
   A) Stridor
   B) Wheezing
   C) Rhonchi
   D) Crackles

6. Which of the following is the first-line treatment for a patient experiencing a seizure?
   A) Administer a benzodiazepine
   B) Insert an oral airway
   C) Protect from injury
   D) Begin CPR

7. The presence of bright red blood in vomit typically suggests what type of condition?
   A) Peptic ulcer
   B) Gastritis
   C) Esophageal varices
   D) Gastroenteritis

8. Which of the following symptoms is most indicative of meningitis in adults?
   A) Headache
   B) Nausea and vomiting
   C) Neck stiffness
   D) High fever

9. A patient with a history of chronic obstructive pulmonary disease (COPD) is most likely to present with which symptom?
   A) Chronic productive cough
   B) Wheezing
   C) Shortness of breath
   D) All of the above

10. A patient who overdosed on a narcotic will likely exhibit which of the following symptoms?
    A) Hypertension and tachycardia
    B) Dilated pupils and agitation
    C) Respiratory depression and pinpoint pupils
    D) Hyperactivity and hallucinations

11. A patient experiencing heat stroke will likely have which of the following vital signs?
    A) Low heart rate and high blood pressure
    B) High heart rate and high blood pressure
    C) Low heart rate and low blood pressure
    D) High heart rate and low blood pressure

12. Which is the most common sign of a urinary tract infection?
    A) Hematuria
    B) Dysuria
    C) Lower back pain
    D) Fever

13. The term "agonal breathing" refers to which of the following?
    A) Normal, regular breaths
    B) Rapid, shallow breathing
    C) Gasping, irregular breaths
    D) Deep, slow breaths

14. In anaphylaxis, which of the following interventions should be initiated first?
    A) Administer epinephrine
    B) Administer antihistamine
    C) Establish an airway
    D) Begin CPR

15. Which of the following is not a symptom of opiate withdrawal?
    A) Dilated pupils
    B) Vomiting and diarrhoea
    C) Agitation
    D) Respiratory depression

Trauma

1. What's the most common type of shock in a trauma patient?
   A) Septic shock
   B) Cardiogenic shock
   C) Hypovolemic shock
   D) Neurogenic shock

2. In managing a suspected spinal injury patient, which of the following is the best immobilization method?
   A) Soft collar
   B) Hard collar and spine board
   C) Manual stabilization
   D) Sandbags on either side of the head

3. What is the priority in managing a trauma patient with multiple injuries?
   A) Controlling bleeding
   B) Stabilizing fractures
   C) Checking airway, breathing, and circulation
   D) Assessing the level of consciousness

4. Which type of injury is most likely to cause a tension pneumothorax?
   A) Blunt force trauma to the chest
   B) Penetrating chest wound
   C) Fractured ribs
   D) Pulmonary contusion

5. How should an impaled object in the chest be managed?
   A) Remove it immediately
   B) Stabilize it in place
   C) Apply direct pressure around it
   D) Cover with a wet dressing

6. A patient with a severe head injury presents with uneven pupil sizes. This condition is known as?
   A) Anisocoria
   B) Mydriasis
   C) Miosis
   D) Anisometropia

7. Which of the following is not a common sign of a pelvic fracture?
   A) Pain and tenderness in the pelvic area
   B) Instability of the pelvic ring
   C) Deformity of the pelvic area
   D) Immediate loss of consciousness

8. In trauma patients, the 'Golden Hour' refers to the?
   A) The hour immediately after the injury
   B) The first hour of surgery
   C) The hour after arrival at the hospital
   D) The first hour of rehabilitation

9. The term 'evisceration' refers to which of the following?
   A) Fracture of a bone
   B) Dislocation of a joint
   C) Protrusion of an organ through a wound
   D) Deep cut in the skin

10. Which is the best position for a patient with a suspected hip fracture?
    A) Lying flat on the back
    B) Lying on the injured side
    C) Lying on the uninjured side
    D) Legs straight and together

11. A flail chest occurs when?
    A) Three or more adjacent ribs are fractured in two or more places
    B) The sternum is fractured
    C) A single rib is fractured in two places
    D) The chest wall muscles are torn

12. Which of the following is not a common cause of abdominal trauma?
    A) Motor vehicle accidents
    B) Falls from a height
    C) Penetrating injuries
    D) Hypothermia

13. What is the most common type of burn?
    A) Chemical burn
    B) Electrical burn
    C) Thermal burn
    D) Radiation burn

14. In a patient with a suspected fracture, which of the following should be assessed first?
    A) Pain
    B) Deformity
    C) Circulation
    D) Range of motion

15. The Glasgow Coma Scale is used to assess?
    A) Severity of a head injury
    B) Level of consciousness
    C) Memory loss
    D) Both A and B

Special Populations

1. Geriatric patients often present "atypical" symptoms of severe conditions. Which of the following is a joint atypical presentation in older people?
   A) Chest pain from a heart attack
   B) Abdominal pain for appendicitis
   C) Altered mental status for urinary tract infection
   D) Shortness of breath for asthma

2. What is the main challenge with pediatric airway management?
   A) Children's airways are more flexible
   B) Children's airways are proportionally smaller
   C) Children are more prone to hypoxia
   D) All of the above

3. Pregnant patients should be transported in what position to prevent vena cava compression?
   A) Supine
   B) Left lateral decubitus
   C) Right lateral decubitus
   D) Prone

4. Which of the following changes occurs in the respiratory system of a pregnant woman?
   A) Increased tidal volume
   B) Decreased oxygen consumption
   C) Decreased respiratory rate
   D) Increased residual volume

5. When performing CPR on an infant, you should compress the chest:
   A) With two hands
   B) With one hand
   C) With two fingers
   D) With the heel of one hand

6. A neonate's pulse rate is typically:
   A) Slower than an adult's pulse rate
   B) The same as an adult's pulse rate
   C) Faster than an adult's pulse rate
   D) Variable and does not follow a specific pattern

7. Why is hypothermia a common problem in neonates?
   A) They have a high surface area to volume ratio
   B) They lack subcutaneous fat
   C) They have an underdeveloped thermoregulatory system
   D) All of the above

8. When assessing an elderly patient, which of the following factors should be considered?
   A) Presence of multiple medical conditions
   B) Use of multiple medications
   C) Potential for atypical presentations of illness
   D) All of the above

9. What is the most common cause of seizures in children?
   A) Epilepsy
   B) Brain tumour
   C) Febrile seizures
   D) Head injury

10. Which of the following is a typical characteristic of the geriatric population?
   A) They have the same physiological response to illness or injury as younger adults.
   B) They experience pain less intensely than younger adults.
   C) They often have multiple chronic conditions.
   D) They have a faster metabolic rate than younger adults.

EMS Operations

1. What is the primary objective of EMS systems?
   A) Treat patients on the scene
   B) Provide rapid transport to the hospital
   C) Provide care to critically injured patients
   D) Enable patients to reach definitive care

2. What is the goal of an incident command system (ICS)?
   A) Ensure the safety of responders, patients, and the public
   B) Stabilize the incident
   C) Provide for the orderly transfer of personnel and equipment
   D) All of the above

3. During a multiple-casualty incident, what is the first step for an EMT?
   A) Start treating the most critically injured patient
   B) Begin rapid extrication of all patients
   C) Implement the incident command system
   D) Identify all patients at the scene

4. What is the goal of triage during a multiple-casualty incident?
   A) To provide immediate treatment to all patients
   B) To identify the most seriously injured patients
   C) To do the most good for the most people
   D) To transport patients to the hospital as quickly as possible

5. When responding to a hazardous materials incident, the EMT's first concern should be:
   A) Identifying the substance involved
   B) Ensuring their safety and that of the crew
   C) Treating patients at the scene
   D) Notifying the hospital of potential contamination

6. During a terrorist incident, the primary role of an EMT is to:
   A) Identify the perpetrators
   B) Secure the crime scene
   C) Provide care to the injured
   D) Document the incident

7. In a mass-casualty incident, the process of identifying the strategy for the most significant positive impact for the most people is called:
   A) Resource allocation
   B) Triage
   C) Scene size-up
   D) Decontamination

8. Which of the following is part of the ongoing assessment of a scene during EMS operations?
   A) Monitor scene safety
   B) Continually reassess the number of patients
   C) Evaluate the need for additional resources
   D) All of the above

9. What should an EMT do upon arrival at a scene where violence may be ongoing?
   A) Enter immediately and begin patient care
   B) Wait for law enforcement to secure the scene
   C) Begin triage immediately
   D) Enter with caution and attempt to locate the perpetrator

10. When should the use of lights and sirens be considered in ambulance operations?
   A) When the patient's condition is life-threatening
   B) Anytime the ambulance is on the road
   C) When responding to all emergency calls
   D) When the traffic is heavy and causing delays

11. Which of the following is a role of an EMT in air medical transport?
   A) Fly the helicopter
   B) Communicate with air traffic control
   C) Prepare the landing zone
   D) Provide in-flight patient care

12. What is an EMT's role at a crime scene?
   A) Investigate the crime
   B) Protect evidence while providing patient care
   C) Interview witnesses
   D) Apprehend the suspect

13. What does the term "resource management" in EMS operations refer to?
   A) The process of ordering and restocking medical supplies
   B) The management of an EMT's time and energy during a shift
   C) The allocation and coordination of resources during an incident
   D) The management of the EMS agency's budget and finances

14. What is the primary goal of rehabilitation during EMS operations?
   A) To return injured employees to work
   B) To provide rest and recovery to responders during prolonged incidents
   C) To treat and release patients at the scene
   D) To help patients recover from their injuries or illness

15. When transporting a patient to the hospital, which of the following should be prioritized?
   A) Comfortable ride for the patient
   B) Rapid transport, regardless of the patient's condition
   C) Safe and efficient transport based on the patient's condition
   D) Use of lights and sirens to expedite transport

ANSWER KEY

Airway Management

1. Answer: **C)** Head Tilt-Chin Lift
    Reason: The Head Tilt-Chin Lift method is used to open the airway in an unconscious patient without suspected spinal injury. The other options are techniques used in different scenarios or incorrect ones.
2. Answer: **C)** Circulation
    Reason: In the ABCs of emergency medicine, "C" stands for circulation. This mnemonic helps medical professionals remember the correct sequence for life-saving interventions: Airway, Breathing, and Circulation.
3. Answer: **C)** Protecting the airway
    Reason: The primary purpose of the oropharyngeal airway (OP**A)** is to keep the tongue from blocking the upper airway, thereby protecting it.
4. Answer: **B)** Use of accessory muscles
    Reason: Using accessory muscles to breathe is usually a sign of respiratory distress, not adequate breathing.
5. Answer: **B)** Oropharyngeal airway (OPA)
    Reason: An oropharyngeal airway (OP**A)** should not be used in conscious patients as it may cause gagging or vomiting.
6. Answer: **A)** 5 seconds
    Reason: Suctioning should be quick and should not last longer than 5 seconds to minimize oxygen deprivation.
7. Answer: **C)** Recovery Position
    Reason: The recovery position helps keep the airway clear by allowing fluids to drain from the mouth, particularly useful in unconscious patients without suspected spinal injury.
8. Answer: **C)** Need for suctioning
    Reason: Suctioning can be performed without endotracheal intubation. The other options are typical indications for this procedure.
9. Answer: **C)** Suction the airway
    Reason: Gurgling sounds usually indicate the presence of fluid in the airway, and suctioning is the appropriate method to clear it.
10. Answer: **C)** End-tidal CO2
    Reason: Capnography is a monitoring tool used to assess ventilation by measuring the concentration of CO2 at the end of exhalation (end-tidal CO2).
11. Answer: **C)** 30:2
    Reason: The recommended ratio of compressions to breaths for a lone rescuer performing CPR on an adult is 30 compressions to 2 breaths.
12. Answer: **B)** A conscious patient with a gag reflex
    Reason: A nasopharyngeal airway (NP**A)** is often tolerated by conscious patients with gag reflexes. It is contraindicated in patients with suspected or known nasal fractures.
13. Answer: **B)** To prevent gastric contents from entering the lungs
    Reason: Cricoid pressure is used during endotracheal intubation primarily to avoid regurgitating gastric contents, reducing the risk of aspiration.
14. Answer: **B)** Nasopharyngeal airway (NPA)
    Reason: A nasopharyngeal airway (NP**A)** is generally contraindicated in patients with suspected basal skull fractures due to the potential for the tube to enter the cranial vault through the fracture site.
15. Answer: **A)** It extends from the corner of the mouth to the earlobe.

Reason: The correct size of an oropharyngeal airway (OP**A)** should extend from the corner of the mouth to the earlobe. This length generally allows the OPA to maintain an open airway without causing unnecessary trauma or discomfort.

Patient Assessment

1. Answer: **D)** Checking responsiveness
   Reason: The primary survey begins by checking the patient's responsiveness, often using the AVPU scale (Alert, Verbal, Pain, Unresponsive).

2. Answer: **B)** Symptoms, Allergies, Medication, Past medical history, Last oral intake, Events leading up to present illness
   Reason: In the EMT patient assessment, SAMPLE stands for Symptoms, Allergies, Medication, Past medical history, Last oral intake, and Events leading up to the present illness.

3. Answer: **B)** Secondary Survey
   Reason: The Secondary Survey includes a detailed history and physical exam after the Primary Survey has identified and managed all immediate life threats.

4. Answer: **D)** Blood glucose level
   Reason: While blood glucose levels can be significant in specific medical emergencies, they are not considered a traditional vital sign. EMTs commonly assess blood pressure, heart rate, and respiratory rate as part of their patient assessment.

5. Answer: **B)** To determine the severity of traumatic brain injury
   Reason: The Glasgow Coma Scale is primarily used to assess the severity of a traumatic brain injury, including evaluating consciousness and motor and verbal responses.

6. Answer: **B)** Trauma patients with significant mechanisms of injury
   Reason: The Rapid Trauma Assessment is typically conducted during the Primary Survey on trauma patients with an essential means of damage or if the patient's level of consciousness or vital signs is abnormal.

7. Answer: **A)** Onset, Provocation, Quality, Region/Radiation, Severity, Time
   Reason: OPQRST is a mnemonic medical professional use to remember the essential aspects of symptom history taking in patients. It stands for Onset, Provocation, Quality, Region/Radiation, Severity, and Time.

8. Answer: **C)** Blood pressure
   Reason: In pediatric patients, blood pressure is typically the last vital sign to change in response to shock or illness. Pediatric patients can maintain their blood pressure until their condition is critical.

9. Answer: **B)** Inadequate breathing
   Reason: Cyanosis, a bluish discoloration of the skin or mucous membranes, is often a sign of inadequate oxygenation or poor circulation, which can be due to impaired breathing.

10. Answer: **D)** Exacerbation
    Reason: In the PASTE acronym, "E" stands for Exacerbation. The full acronym stands for Provocation or Palliation, Associated chest pain, Sputum production, Talking tiredness (or dyspnea), and Exacerbation.

11. Answer: **D)** Regardless of the patient's mental status
    Reason: A detailed physical exam should be conducted on all patients, regardless of the patient's mental status. It provides additional information and may help to uncover hidden injuries or conditions.

12. Answer: **A)** Tenderness, Instability, Crepitus
    Reason: PITCO is a mnemonic for musculoskeletal assessment. TIC stands for Tenderness, Instability, and Crepitus.

13. Answer: **C)** One-sided weakness or facial drooping
    Reason: One-sided weakness or facial drooping are classic signs of a possible stroke and should prompt immediate action by the EMT to ensure rapid transport and treatment.

14. Answer: **C)** Detecting any areas of pain, distention, or rigidity
    Reason: In a rapid trauma assessment, the EMT's palpation of the abdomen is primarily to detect any areas of pain, expansion, or rigidity which can be indicative of internal injuries.

Medical Emergencies

Medical Emergencies

1. Answer: **C)** Oxygen
   Reason: Oxygen is usually administered first to increase the oxygen supply to the myocardium, which can help minimize damage from a heart attack.
2. Answer: **C)** Tremors and weakness
   Reason: Hypoglycemia, or low blood sugar, can cause various symptoms, including tremors, weakness, confusion, and loss of consciousness.
3. Answer: **B)** Sudden loss of consciousness
   Reason: A syncopal episode, or fainting, is characterized by a sudden, temporary loss of consciousness, usually related to insufficient blood flow to the brain.
4. Answer: **C)** Check airway, breathing, and circulation
   Reason: An EMT's priority is always to check the airway, breathing, and circulation (ABCs) to ensure the patient's vital functions are stable before administering medications.
5. Answer: **B)** Wheezing
   Reason: Wheezing, a high-pitched whistling sound caused by narrowed airways, is a common sign of an asthma attack.
6. Answer: **C)** Protect from injury
   Reason: The priority in managing a patient experiencing a seizure is to protect them from injury by moving surrounding objects out of the way and padding the patient's head.
7. Answer: **C)** Esophageal varices
   Reason: Bright red blood in vomit often indicates esophageal varices, where the veins in the oesophagus burst due to high pressure, though other conditions can also cause this symptom.
8. Answer: **C)** Neck stiffness
   Reason: While all the options can be symptoms of meningitis, neck stiffness or nuchal rigidity is a classic sign of meningitis in adults.
9. Answer: **D)** All of the above
   Reason: Patients with COPD often present with all these symptoms - chronic productive cough, wheezing, and shortness of breath - as part of their chronic condition.
10. Answer: **C)** Respiratory depression and pinpoint pupils
    Reason: Narcotic overdose commonly leads to respiratory depression, miosis (pinpoint pupils), and other symptoms such as altered mental status.
11. Answer: **D)** High heart rate and low blood pressure
    Reason: A patient experiencing heat stroke typically presents with tachycardia (high heart rate) and hypotension (low blood pressure) due to dehydration and the body's response to heat.
12. Answer: **B)** Dysuria.
    Reason: Dysuria refers to painful or difficult urination, which is a frequent symptom experienced by individuals with a UTI..
13. Answer: **C)** Gasping, irregular breaths
    Reason: Agonal breathing refers to gasping, irregular breaths and is often a sign of severe illness or near death.
14. Answer: **A)** Administer epinephrine
    Reason: In anaphylaxis, administering epinephrine is the first and most crucial intervention.
15. Answer: **D)** Respiratory depression
    Reason: Respiratory depression is a common symptom of opiate use, not withdrawal. Symptoms of opiate withdrawal include dilated pupils, vomiting, diarrhoea, agitation, and other flu-like symptoms.

Trauma

1. Answer: **C)** Hypovolemic shock
    Reason: Hypovolemic shock results from significant blood loss and is the most common shock in trauma patients.
2. Answer: **B)** Hard collar and spine board
    Reason: A stiff collar and spine board offer the most effective immobilization for suspected spinal injuries to prevent further damage.
3. Answer: **C)** Checking airway, breathing, and circulation
    Reason: The priority in trauma management is always to check the airway, breathing, and circulation (ABCs) to ensure the patient's vital functions are stable.
4. Answer: **B)** Penetrating chest wound
    Reason: Tension pneumothorax is commonly caused by a penetrating chest wound, which allows air to enter the pleural space and cannot escape, leading to increased pressure on the lungs and heart.
5. Answer: **B)** Stabilize it in place
    Reason: An impaled object should be stabilized and not removed at the scene, as removal can cause additional injury and bleeding.
6. Answer: **A)** Anisocoria
    Reason: Anisocoria refers to a condition in which the patient's pupils are different sizes, which can signify a severe head injury.
7. Answer: **D)** Immediate loss of consciousness
    Reason: Immediate loss of consciousness is not typically associated with a pelvic fracture, while pain, tenderness, instability, and deformity in the pelvic area are common signs.
8. Answer: **A)** The hour immediately after injury
    Reason: The 'Golden Hour' in trauma refers to the hour immediately after injury, a critical period during which prompt medical treatment significantly increases a patient's chance of survival.
9. Answer: **C)** Protrusion of an organ through a wound
    Reason: Evisceration refers to the protrusion of an organ through a wound, typically in the abdomen.
10. Answer: **A)** Lying flat on the back
    Reason: A patient with a suspected hip fracture should be placed flat on their back, with the injured leg slightly bent and supported to minimize pain.
11. Answer: **A)** Three or more adjacent ribs are fractured in two or more places
    Reason: A flail chest occurs when three or more adjacent ribs are fractured in two or more locations, causing the chest wall to become unstable.
12. Answer: **D)** Hypothermia
    Reason: Hypothermia is not a common cause of abdominal trauma. Motor vehicle accidents falls, and penetrating injuries are common causes.
13. Answer: **C)** Thermal burn
    Reason: Thermal burns, which result from exposure to flames or hot objects, are the most common type of burn.
14. Answer: **C)** Circulation
    Reason: In a patient with a suspected fracture, the first thing to assess is circulation. If blood flow is compromised, it could lead to tissue death and permanent damage.
15. Answer: **D)** Both A and B
    Reason: The Glasgow Coma Scale is a tool used to assess the severity of a head injury and the patient's level of consciousness.

Special Populations

1. Answer: **C)** Altered mental status for urinary tract infection
   Reason: Geriatric patients often present "atypical" symptoms, such as altered mental status due to a urinary tract infection, which is not typical in younger patients.
2. Answer: **D)** All of the above
   Reason: Pediatric airway management can be challenging due to children's smaller, more flexible airways and increased susceptibility to hypoxia.
3. Answer: **B)** Left lateral decubitus
   Reason: Pregnant patients should be transported to the left lateral decubitus position to prevent compression of the vena cava.
4. Answer: **A)** Increased tidal volume
   Reason: During pregnancy, a woman's tidal volume (the air moved into and out of the lungs during each respiratory cycle) increases.
5. Answer: **C)** With two fingers
   Reason: When CPR on an infant, the chest should be compressed gently with two fingers.
6. Answer: **C)** Faster than an adult's pulse rate
   Reason: A neonate (an infant less than a month ol**D)** typically has a faster pulse rate than an adult.
7. Answer: **D)** All of the above
   Reason: Neonates are prone to hypothermia due to their high surface area-to-volume ratio, lack of subcutaneous fat, and underdeveloped thermoregulatory system.
8. Answer: **D)** All of the above
   Reason: When assessing an elderly patient, you should consider multiple medical conditions, multiple medications, and the potential for atypical illness presentations.
9. Answer: **C)** Febrile seizures
   Reason: Febrile seizures, triggered by high body temperature, are the most common cause of seizures in children.
10. Answer: **C)** They often have multiple chronic conditions.
    Reason: Geriatric patients often have multiple chronic conditions, complicating their medical management and response to illness or injury.

EMS Operations

1. Answer: **D)** Enable patients to reach definitive care. The main objective of EMS is to provide immediate care and transport patients to standard care in the shortest possible time.
2. Answer: **D)** All of the above. ICS provides a systematic tool for the command, control, and coordination of emergency response, aiming to ensure safety, stabilize the incident, and enable the orderly transfer of resources.
3. Answer: **C)** Implement the incident command system. Establishing an incident command system should be the first step to managing resources and coordinating the response effectively.
4. Answer: **C)** To do the most good for the most people. Triage aims to prioritize patients based on the severity of their condition and the available resources to benefit the most significant number of patients.
5. Answer: **B)** Ensuring their safety and that of the crew. Safety is always the primary concern in hazardous materials incidents.
6. Answer: **C)** Provide care to the injured. The primary role of an EMT during any emergency, including a terrorist incident, is to provide care to the wounded while ensuring personal safety.
7. Answer: **B)** Triage. In a mass-casualty incident, triage is the process used to sort patients based on the severity of their condition to maximize the number of survivors.
8. Answer: **D)** All of the above. The ongoing scene assessment involves continuously monitoring scene safety, reassessing patient numbers, and evaluating the need for additional resources.
9. Answer: **B)** Wait for law enforcement to secure the scene. An EMT should only enter a potentially violent location once law enforcement has confirmed it.
10. Answer: **A)** When the patient's condition is life-threatening. The use of lights and sirens should be limited to situations where the patient's condition is life-threatening and rapid transport is necessary.
11. Answer: **C)** Prepare the landing zone. The EMT's role in air medical transport typically includes preparing the landing zone and providing ground support.
12. Answer: **B)** Protect evidence while providing patient care. While the primary role of an EMT is patient care, they should also aim to preserve evidence when possible.
13. Answer: **C)** The allocation and coordination of resources during an incident. Resource management involves effectively allocating and coordinating resources, including personnel, equipment, and vehicles, during an incident.
14. Answer: **B)** To provide rest and recovery to responders during prolonged incidents. Rehabilitation in the context of EMS operations refers to activities aimed at maintaining the well-being of responders during incidents, particularly those of long duration.
15. Answer: **C)** Safe and efficient transport based on the patient's condition. The priority during patient transport should always be safety and efficiency, considering the patient's specific medical needs.

QUESTIONS & ANSWERS

Airway Management

Question: What is the primary objective of airway management in an emergency medical scenario?
Answer: The primary goal of airway management is to establish and maintain a clear and unobstructed passage for air to move in and out of the lungs. This entails preventing obstructions, ensuring adequate oxygen supply, and removing carbon dioxide. The ability to breathe effectively is fundamental to life, and any compromise can lead to hypoxia, hypercapnia, and other severe complications. In an emergency, airway management thus becomes a top priority.

Question: What is a 'patent airway'?
Answer: In medical terminology, a 'patent airway' is an airway that is open and free from obstructions, permitting air to pass freely from the exterior environment to the alveoli in the lungs. This involves an unimpeded path from the nostrils and mouth, through the pharynx and larynx, down the trachea, and into the bronchi and lungs. Ensuring a patent airway is critical in emergency medical care to facilitate proper respiration.

Question: What artificial airways are commonly used in emergency medical services (EMS)?
Answer: In EMS, oropharyngeal airways (OPAs) and nasopharyngeal airways (NPAs) are artificial airways commonly used to maintain a patient's airway. These devices are designed to bypass upper airway obstructions, often caused by the tongue or other soft tissues, and create a safe and clear route for air to flow into the lungs. While OPAs and NPAs serve similar purposes, they differ in insertion and appropriate patient conditions.

Question: Differentiate between ventilation and respiration.
Answer: Ventilation and respiration, though related, are distinct processes within the broader concept of breathing. Ventilation is a mechanical process that involves the physical movement of air in and out of the lungs, facilitated by the expansion and contraction of the chest cavity. On the other hand, respiration is a chemical process where oxygen from inhaled air is exchanged for carbon dioxide in the blood at the alveolar level. Ventilation is about transporting air, while respiration concerns the exchange of gases.

Question: What is the 'head-tilt chin-lift maneuver, and when is it utilized?
Answer: The 'head-tilt chin-lift is an essential manual maneuver used in unconscious patients to clear the airway of obstructions and facilitate breathing. The patient's head is tilted backward while the chin is lifted upward. This action pulls the tongue away from the back of the throat, opening the airway. However, it's critical to note that this technique should only be used when there's no suspicion of cervical spine injury, as it could potentially exacerbate such injuries.

Question: Why would the 'jaw-thrust' manoeuvre be preferred over the 'head-tilt chin-lift'?
Answer: The 'jaw-thrust' maneuver is preferred over the 'head-tilt chin-lift when a cervical spine injury is suspected or known. The 'jaw-thrust' technique, which involves manually displacing the jaw forward without moving the neck, helps maintain the airway's patency while minimizing potential spinal movement, reducing the risk of causing or exacerbating spinal injuries.

Question: What is the purpose of suctioning in airway management?
Answer: Suctioning is crucial in airway management, mainly when obstructions occur. Obstructions can include fluids such as blood, vomit, or other foreign material that impedes air passage. By removing these obstructions, suctioning helps maintain a patent airway and prevent aspiration, which can lead to severe complications like pneumonia or a lung abscess.

Question: What is 'bag-valve mask' (BVM) ventilation, and in which situations is it used?
Answer: Bag-valve mask (BVM) ventilation manually assists or replaces a patient's breathing. It involves using a handheld device to push air into the lungs and is used when a patient is in respiratory distress, not breathing effectively, or not breathing at all. This technique can provide a higher concentration of oxygen and can be life-saving in critical situations such as cardiac or respiratory arrest.

Question: How does a laryngoscope assist in airway management?
Answer: A laryngoscope is a tool used in the endotracheal intubation procedure. It helps visualize the vocal cords and guides the endotracheal tube into the trachea, thus establishing a definitive airway. By allowing direct visualization, it significantly reduces the risks of incorrect tube placement and related complications.

Question: What is the purpose of performing a cricothyrotomy in airway management?
Answer: A cricothyrotomy, sometimes referred to as a 'surgical airway,' is a procedure performed when conventional methods of airway management have failed or are not suitable. The process involves making an incision through the skin and cricothyroid membrane in the neck to establish an airway, allowing air to be delivered directly to the lungs. It's a last-resort procedure used in life-threatening emergencies.

Question: How can capnography assist in airway management?
Answer: Capnography is a tool that measures the amount of carbon dioxide (CO_2) in the air a person exhales, termed end-tidal CO_2 ($EtCO_2$). It's a valuable resource in airway management as it provides real-time feedback about ventilation effectiveness and the patient's metabolic and circulatory status. For instance, it can confirm successful endotracheal intubation, monitor the quality of CPR, and detect changes in a patient's condition, such as hypoventilation or hyperventilation.

Question: What is a supraglottic airway device, and when might it be used?
Answer: A supraglottic airway device is an airway tool placed within the upper airway (above the vocal cords) to facilitate ventilation. Examples include the laryngeal mask airway (LMA) and King LT airway. These devices are often used when endotracheal intubation is unsuccessful, contraindicated, or when the provider does not have the necessary skills or equipment to perform intubation.

Question: How does pulse oximetry assist in airway management?
Answer: Pulse oximetry is a non-invasive monitoring tool that measures the blood's oxygen saturation level (SpO_2). It provides continuous, immediate feedback about a patient's oxygenation status directly related to airway patency and ventilation effectiveness. Early identification of hypoxia, before it becomes clinically evident, can guide interventions and prevent severe complications.

Question: What are the indications for rapid sequence intubation (RSI)?
Answer: Rapid sequence intubation (RSI) is an advanced airway management technique used when a patient's airway is compromised and they're unable to maintain adequate ventilation and oxygenation. It involves the administration of a rapid-onset sedative and a neuromuscular blocking agent to facilitate endotracheal intubation. Indications for RSI include respiratory failure, shock, severe head injury, and other severe illnesses requiring immediate airway control.

Question: What role does a nasopharyngeal airway (NPA) play in managing a patient's airway?
Answer: A nasopharyngeal airway (NPA) is a flexible tube inserted into the nose that extends to the level of the oropharynx. It helps maintain an open airway by preventing soft tissues (like the tongue) from obstructing the pharynx. NPAs are often used in semi-conscious or unconscious patients with an intact gag reflex, where an oropharyngeal airway could cause vomiting or aspiration. They also benefit patients with oral injuries or obstructions that prevent using an oropharyngeal airway.

Patient Assessment

Question: What are the essential components of the primary assessment in an EMS setting?
Answer: The primary assessment in an EMS setting consists of immediate checks to identify and manage life-threatening conditions. These components include scene safety assessment, general impression, assessing mental status (using AVPU or alertness, voice, pain, unresponsiveness), airway assessment, breathing assessment, circulation assessment, and determining patient priority for transport and treatment.

Question: How do EMTs assess a patient's level of consciousness?
Answer: EMTs typically assess a patient's level of consciousness using the AVPU scale. This acronym stands for Alert, Verbal response, Painful response, and Unresponsive. The patient's response to various stimuli, such as questions or gentle prodding, helps determine their consciousness level and provides valuable information about their neurological status.

Question: What does the SAMPLE history include?
Answer: The SAMPLE history is a mnemonic used to gather essential information about a patient's medical background. It stands for Symptoms, Allergies, Medications, Past medical history, Last oral intake, and Events leading up to the present illness or injury. This information helps guide further assessment and treatment and provides valuable context to healthcare providers.

Question: Why is it vital to assess a patient's skin colour, temperature, and condition?
Answer: Evaluating a patient's skin color, temperature, and condition provides clues to their health. Pale or bluish skin may indicate poor circulation or hypoxia. Warm and dry skin might be expected, while cool and clammy skin could signal shock or anxiety. Assessing these factors gives healthcare providers insight into blood flow, hydration, and the body's overall physiological status.

Question: What is the purpose of the secondary assessment in EMS?
Answer: The secondary assessment follows the primary evaluation and focuses on a detailed patient examination, targeting specific injuries or illnesses. It typically involves a head-to-toe physical examination and vital signs measurement and may include focused history taking. The secondary assessment allows for a more comprehensive understanding of the patient's condition, leading to more effective treatment and care.

Question: How is pain evaluated in a patient assessment?
Answer: Pain is often assessed using a subjective scale, such as a numeric rating scale where patients rate their pain from 0 (no pain) to 10 (worst pain imaginable). EMTs may also ask the patient to describe the quality, location, onset, duration, and factors that alleviate or exacerbate the pain. This assessment helps in understanding the underlying cause and guides pain management strategies.

Question: What are the normal ranges for vital signs like blood pressure, pulse, and respiration?
Answer: Normal vital signs vary based on age, sex, weight, exercise capacity, and overall health. Generally, a normal blood pressure range is systolic 90-120 mm Hg and diastolic 60-80 mm Hg; a normal pulse rate is 60-100 beats per minute, and normal respiration is 12-20 breaths per minute. Noting deviations from these ranges may indicate underlying health problems.

Question: What's the importance of the "Glasgow Coma Scale" in patient assessment?
Answer: The Glasgow Coma Scale (GCS) is a standardized tool used to assess a patient's level of consciousness by evaluating eye, verbal, and motor responses. Scores range from 3 (deep unconsciousness) to 15 (full alertness), quantifying a patient's neurological function. This assessment can guide treatment decisions and is valuable in monitoring patient condition changes.

Question: When would an EMT perform a "focused physical exam"?
Answer: A focused physical exam is conducted when a patient has sustained specific injuries or is experiencing a localized complaint. Unlike a complete head-to-toe examination, this assessment zeroes in on a particular body system or part. For example, in the case of a suspected fracture, the EMT would focus on the affected limb's examination.

Question: What is the significance of Pupil Assessment in a neurological examination?

Answer: Pupil assessment evaluates pupil size, shape, and reaction to light. It's a crucial part of a neurological examination as changes in these aspects can signal underlying brain injury, drug use, eye trauma, or other neurological conditions. Consistent monitoring can also detect changes in a patient's neurological status over time.

Question: How does the "OPQRST" mnemonic aid in pain assessment?

Answer: The OPQRST mnemonic helps EMTs systematically assess a patient's pain by asking about Onset, Provocation or Palliation, Quality, Region and Radiation, Severity, and Timing. This detailed approach offers insight into the nature and possible cause of the pain, allowing for more targeted treatment and care.

Question: What are the critical aspects of assessing a patient's breathing?

Answer: Assessing a patient's breathing involves evaluating the rate, rhythm, depth, and quality of breaths. It includes observing chest rise, listening for breath sounds, and feeling for air movement. Abnormalities like wheezing, shallow breathing, or asymmetrical chest expansion can indicate respiratory issues that require immediate intervention.

Question: Why is continuous monitoring essential in patient assessment?

Answer: Continuous monitoring allows healthcare providers to promptly detect changes in a patient's condition, enabling immediate intervention. It helps evaluate the effectiveness of treatments given and aids in making decisions about further treatment plans.

Question: What role does a patient's medical history play in EMS patient assessment?

Answer: A patient's medical history provides valuable information about existing medical conditions, past surgeries, allergies, and medications that might influence their health status. It can also offer clues about the cause of the present illness or injury and guide the EMT in making treatment decisions.

Question: How is the reassessment phase of patient assessment significant in EMS?

Answer: The reassessment phase in patient assessment involves repeating the primary and secondary evaluations to identify changes in the patient's condition. It helps evaluate the treatments' effectiveness and guides further treatment decisions. Reassessment should occur regularly during the patient's entire care, ensuring optimal care.

Medical emergencies

QUESTION: What is a myocardial infarction, and how is it treated in the field?
ANSWER: A myocardial infarction, commonly known as a heart attack, is a medical emergency where blood flow to part of the heart gets blocked, causing damage to the heart muscle. If prescribed, EMTs can administer aspirin to thin the blood and nitroglycerin, closely monitor the patient's vital signs, and provide oxygen if needed. Prompt transportation to the hospital is crucial, as definitive care is required.

QUESTION: Describe the signs and symptoms of a stroke.
ANSWER: Stroke symptoms may include sudden numbness or weakness, particularly on one side of the body, confusion or trouble speaking, visual impairments, difficulty walking or maintaining balance, and a sudden, severe headache. Rapid assessment and transport to a stroke centre are vital, as timely intervention can minimize long-term disabilities.

QUESTION: How do EMTs assess and manage a diabetic emergency?
ANSWER: In a diabetic emergency, EMTs assess the patient's blood sugar level, if possible, look for medical identification, and ask about any history of diabetes. Treatment may include administering oral glucose if the patient is conscious and can swallow. Monitoring vital signs and providing supportive care during transport is also essential.

QUESTION: What is anaphylaxis, and how is it managed in the prehospital setting?
ANSWER: Anaphylaxis is a severe, life-threatening allergic reaction that can occur rapidly. Symptoms may include difficulty breathing, swelling of the face and throat, hives, and a rapid or weak pulse. If prescribed, EMTs may administer epinephrine via an auto-injector, provide supplemental oxygen, and transport the patient rapidly to the hospital.

QUESTION: What are the primary interventions for a patient experiencing severe asthma symptoms?
ANSWER: For severe asthma symptoms, EMTs would provide high-flow oxygen, encourage the patient to use their prescribed inhaler, assist with the inhaler if necessary, monitor vital signs, and transport quickly. Continuous assessment is crucial, as the patient's condition can deteriorate rapidly.

QUESTION: Describe the general approach to managing a patient with a seizure.
ANSWER: During a seizure, EMTs should focus on protecting the patient from injury by moving objects away from them, maintaining an open airway, and monitoring vital signs. After the seizure, the patient should be placed in recovery, reassured, and transported to the hospital for further evaluation and care.

QUESTION: How is chest pain evaluated and managed in the prehospital setting?
ANSWER: Chest pain evaluation includes assessing the onset, quality, radiation, severity, timing, and associated symptoms. EMTs provide oxygen if needed, administer nitroglycerin and aspirin if prescribed, monitor vital signs, and transport promptly, keeping the receiving facility informed.

QUESTION: What are the common signs and symptoms of congestive heart failure (CHF), and how is it treated in the field?
ANSWER: CHF may present with shortness of breath, chest pain, oedema in the lower extremities, and fatigue. Treatment includes positioning the patient comfortably, often sitting, administering oxygen, possibly assisting with prescribed medications like nitroglycerin, and providing rapid transport to a medical facility.

QUESTION: Describe the management of a patient with suspected hypothermia.
ANSWER: Hypothermia treatment includes removing the patient from the cold environment, protecting them from the wind, insulating them with blankets, applying gentle warmth if possible, and providing careful handling to prevent cardiac irritations. Rapid but gentle transport to a hospital is essential, as aggressive rewarming must be medically supervised.

QUESTION: What is the role of the EMT in managing a psychiatric emergency?
ANSWER: In a psychiatric emergency, the EMT's role is to ensure scene safety, provide a calm and supportive environment, attempt to understand the patient's perception of events and establish trust. Transport to a mental health facility may be required, with continuous observation to ensure patient safety.

QUESTION: What are the signs and symptoms of carbon monoxide poisoning, and how is it managed?
ANSWER: Carbon monoxide poisoning might present with headache, dizziness, weakness, nausea, confusion, chest pain, and unconsciousness. EMTs should remove the patient from the environment, administer high-flow oxygen, monitor vital signs, and provide rapid transport for further medical care.

QUESTION: How do you recognize and treat heat exhaustion in the prehospital setting?
ANSWER: Heat exhaustion can manifest as cool, moist skin, dizziness, headache, nausea, and weakness. Treatment includes moving the patient to a more relaxed environment, providing fluids if they are conscious and can swallow, and offering gentle cooling measures like fans or damp cloths. Transport to the hospital for evaluation is essential.

QUESTION: How is a patient with a suspected opioid overdose treated in the field?
ANSWER: In suspected opioid overdose, signs might include respiratory depression, unconsciousness, pinpoint pupils, and possibly drug paraphernalia presence. Treatment can consist of administering naloxone, providing ventilatory support, closely monitoring vital signs, and transporting to the hospital.

QUESTION: What signs suggest a patient has a panic attack, and how should it be managed?
ANSWER: Panic attacks can present symptoms similar to life-threatening conditions, including chest pain, shortness of breath, and palpitations. EMTs should provide reassurance, encourage slow, controlled breathing, and, if necessary, transport the patient to the hospital for further evaluation to rule out other conditions.

QUESTION: How should an EMT manage a patient presenting with abdominal pain?
ANSWER: Management of abdominal pain includes a thorough assessment to understand the pain's location, quality, severity, associated symptoms, and any relevant medical history. EMTs provide a comfortable position of ease, monitor vital signs, and transport to the hospital for definitive diagnosis and treatment.

QUESTION: What is the initial management of a patient with severe bleeding?
ANSWER: Initial management of severe bleeding involves applying direct pressure with a clean dressing, using a tourniquet if necessary for uncontrolled extremity bleeding, elevating the injury if possible, and providing rapid transport. Continuous monitoring of the patient's status is essential.

QUESTION: Describe the assessment and management of a patient with shortness of breath.
ANSWER: Assessment involves identifying the breath's quality, any associated symptoms, and the patient's medical history. If indicated, EMTs should administer high-flow oxygen, assist with prescribed inhalers or nitroglycerin, monitor vital signs, and provide rapid transport to a medical facility.

QUESTION: How is pain evaluated in the prehospital setting?
ANSWER: Pain is evaluated using the OPQRST acronym: Onset, Provocation/Palliation, Quality, Region/Radiation, Severity, and Time. EMTs should provide comfort measures, administer prescribed or protocol-driven analgesics if indicated, and transport the patient to the hospital for further evaluation.

QUESTION: What is the treatment for a patient experiencing a syncopal episode (fainting)?
ANSWER: Management of syncope involves placing the patient in a supine position to improve blood flow to the brain, monitoring vital signs, identifying potential causes, and providing transport for further evaluation, as the underlying cause could be severe.

QUESTION: How do you manage a patient with a severe headache in the field?
ANSWER: Management of a severe headache involves a thorough assessment, including onset, location, severity, and associated symptoms. Comfort measures, monitoring vital signs, and providing a calm, quiet environment can help. Transport to the hospital is required for further evaluation, as severe conditions like meningitis or a brain aneurysm must be ruled out.

Trauma

QUESTION: What is the primary survey in trauma, and why is it important?
ANSWER: The primary survey in trauma consists of the immediate evaluation and management of life-threatening injuries, including Airway, Breathing, Circulation, Disability, and Exposure (ABCDE). This step-by-step approach ensures the most critical injuries are addressed first.

QUESTION: How do EMTs initially manage a traumatic brain injury?
ANSWER: EMTs should maintain cervical spine immobilization if there is a potential spinal injury, ensure adequate oxygenation, and provide rapid transport. Close monitoring of the patient's level of consciousness, vital signs, and pupillary response is crucial.

QUESTION: Describe the management of a patient with suspected spinal trauma.
ANSWER: Management includes maintaining immobilization, often using a cervical collar and long spine board, monitoring and supporting airway, breathing, and circulation, and transporting promptly to a trauma centre. Regular reassessments are needed to identify any deteriorating neurological function.

QUESTION: What is the initial approach to a patient with a gunshot wound?
ANSWER: The initial approach includes ensuring scene safety, applying direct pressure to control bleeding, treating shock symptoms, protecting the wound with a sterile dressing, and providing prompt transport to a trauma centre.

QUESTION: How should a patient with a suspected fracture be managed in the prehospital setting?
ANSWER: A suspected fracture should be immobilized in the position of comfort or anatomical alignment, pain should be managed, and the patient should be transported for further imaging and definitive care. The distal pulse, motor function, and sensation should be assessed before and after immobilization.

QUESTION: What are the signs and symptoms of a tension pneumothorax, and how is it managed?
ANSWER: Tension pneumothorax might present with severe respiratory distress, decreased or absent lung sounds on one side, tracheal deviation, distended neck veins, and shock. High-flow oxygen, needle decompression by advanced providers, and rapid transport are necessary.

QUESTION: Describe the prehospital management of a patient with burns.
ANSWER: Management of burns includes stopping the burning process, cooling the burn with room temperature water, covering the area with a sterile, non-adhesive dressing, treating for shock, and providing prompt transport. The severity and extent of the burn need to be assessed.

QUESTION: How do you manage a patient with impaled objects following trauma?
ANSWER: Impaled objects should be stabilized in place with bulky dressings and never removed in the field. Control bleeding, treat for shock, and transport promptly. Tetanus prophylaxis and antibiotics will likely be needed.

QUESTION: How should a patient with a possible concussion be managed?
ANSWER: Manage concussion by assessing the patient's neurological status, monitoring for deterioration, and transporting them to a hospital for further evaluation. The patient should avoid activities that might risk a second head injury.

QUESTION: What are the key steps in managing a patient with a pelvic fracture?
ANSWER: A pelvic fracture should be stabilized using a pelvic binder if available, control external bleeding, provide pain relief, and transport with care to a trauma centre. Avoid unnecessary movement of the pelvis to prevent worsening the injury.

QUESTION: What are the signs of peritonitis, and how is it managed in the field?
ANSWER: Peritonitis might present with severe abdominal pain, rigidity, and signs of shock. EMTs should provide a position of comfort, administer oxygen, monitor vital signs, and provide rapid transport to the hospital.

QUESTION: How should a patient with a crush injury be managed in the prehospital setting?
ANSWER: Management includes removing the crushing force if possible and safe, providing pain relief, treating for shock, and transporting promptly. Be alert for signs of crush syndrome, including hyperkalemia and renal failure.

QUESTION: Describe the initial management of a patient with a stab wound.
ANSWER: Initial stab wound management includes controlling bleeding with direct pressure, applying a sterile dressing, and providing rapid transport. Monitor vital signs closely and treat for shock if present.

QUESTION: How do you manage an amputated limb in the field?
ANSWER: Manage an amputated limb by controlling bleeding with a tourniquet or direct pressure, wrapping the amputated part in a sterile dressing, placing it in a plastic bag, and then placing the bag on ice if available. Avoid direct contact of the amputated part with ice. Rapid transport is needed.

QUESTION: What are the signs and symptoms of compartment syndrome, and how is it managed?
ANSWER: Signs of compartment syndrome include severe pain, pallor, pulselessness, paresthesia, and paralysis. EMTs should maintain limb alignment, provide pain relief, and transport promptly. Surgical intervention is required to relieve pressure.

QUESTION: How should a patient with multiple rib fractures be managed?
ANSWER: Management of multiple rib fractures includes providing supplemental oxygen, managing pain, monitoring for complications such as a flail chest or pneumothorax, and prompt transport to a trauma center.

QUESTION: What is the primary concern in a patient with a suspected blast injury?
ANSWER: The primary concern is multiple potential injury sites, including direct blast injuries (lung, ear, and gastrointestinal tract), secondary (penetrating or blunt trauma), tertiary (from being thrown), and quaternary (burns, crush injuries, etc). Rapid assessment and transport are critical.

QUESTION: How should a patient with an open chest wound be managed in the prehospital setting?
ANSWER: An open chest wound should be immediately covered with an occlusive dressing taped on three sides to prevent a tension pneumothorax. Monitor for respiratory distress, manage pain, and provide prompt transport.

QUESTION: How should a patient with hypovolemic shock due to trauma be managed?
ANSWER: Hypovolemic shock should be managed by controlling external bleeding, providing high-flow oxygen, positioning the patient supine, maintaining warmth, and providing rapid transport. Advanced providers may start intravenous fluid resuscitation.

QUESTION: How should a patient with a potential neck injury be managed?
ANSWER: A potential neck injury should be managed by maintaining cervical spine immobilization using a cervical collar, monitoring and supporting the airway, breathing, and circulation, and providing rapid transport to a trauma center.

Special Populations

QUESTION: How does the assessment of a pediatric patient differ from an adult patient?
ANSWER: In pediatric patients, developmental and physiological differences must be taken into account. The approach should be gentle, assessments often must be adapted to the child's age and developmental level, and vital sign ranges vary.

QUESTION: What changes occur in the respiratory system of the elderly, and how might this affect their response to illness or injury?
ANSWER: In older people, respiratory muscles may weaken, lung elasticity may decrease, and cough reflex may diminish. These changes can make elderly patients more susceptible to respiratory diseases and complications, and their recovery may be slower.

QUESTION: How should a patient with suspected dementia be assessed?
ANSWER: Assessment of a patient with suspected dementia should be patient and gentle, using simple language. Information may need to be obtained from family or caregivers. Respond to non-verbal cues, and check for medical ID bracelets or necklaces.

QUESTION: How does pregnancy affect the physiological response to trauma?
ANSWER: Pregnancy can shift organs, increase blood volume, and affect the respiratory system, all of which can change the presentation and progression of trauma. Also, the fetus is at risk, and there's potential for placental abruption or premature labour.

QUESTION: What special considerations are needed for assessing and managing a bariatric patient?
ANSWER: Bariatric patients may require additional personnel for safe handling and transport, have difficulty positioning and breathing, and may have associated health conditions like hypertension or diabetes. Their size may make assessments more challenging.

QUESTION: What factors should be considered when assessing and managing a homeless patient?
ANSWER: Consider the potential for hypothermia or hyperthermia, malnutrition, chronic diseases, mental health disorders, substance abuse, and communicable diseases. The patient may lack access to regular healthcare and medications.

QUESTION: How should a non-English speaking patient be assessed and managed?
ANSWER: Use of an interpreter is ideal. Some agencies have phone translation services. Be patient, and use simple words and non-verbal cues. Always confirm understanding, and avoid using family members as interpreters for complex or sensitive information.

QUESTION: What is unique about the cardiovascular system of a geriatric patient?
ANSWER: Aging leads to stiffening of the vessels, slowing heart rate, and increased risk of hypertension and atherosclerosis. Geriatric patients may also have atypical symptoms of cardiac distress, such as confusion or abdominal pain.

QUESTION: How does an assessment of a neonate differ from an older child?
ANSWER: Neonates have immature systems, are more susceptible to heat loss, and cannot localize infections. Heart rate and respiratory rate are higher. Assessment should be gentle and quick, and parents should be involved when possible.

QUESTION: How should the EMT assess and manage a patient with Down syndrome?
ANSWER: The EMT should be aware of potential congenital heart defects, risk of atlantoaxial instability, and potential communication difficulties. Treat the patient respectfully and patiently, and obtain as much medical history as possible.

QUESTION: What are some common complications of pregnancy that an EMT might encounter?
ANSWER: EMTs might encounter preeclampsia, gestational diabetes, miscarriage, premature labour, or placental abruption. Each presents with different symptoms and needs other management in the field.

QUESTION: What should an EMT consider when dealing with a patient who has a severe intellectual disability?
ANSWER: EMTs should communicate, treat the patient respectfully, involve caregivers in the assessment, and be patient. These individuals may react differently to pain or distress and may have associated medical conditions.

QUESTION: How should a suspected child abuse case be handled in the field?
ANSWER: EMTs should provide medical care for the child, document findings thoroughly, and report suspicions to the appropriate authorities. Don't confront the suspected abuser in the field.

QUESTION: What are common chronic conditions in elderly patients that could affect their management in emergency situations?
ANSWER: Common conditions include cardiac diseases, respiratory diseases, diabetes, dementia, and arthritis. These could affect the presentation and management of acute illnesses or injuries.

QUESTION: What are the unique considerations for trauma in the pregnant patient?
ANSWER: Fetal distress can occur even if the mother seems fine. If possible, the patient should be transported on her left side to prevent supine hypotensive syndrome. Preterm labour and placental abruption are concerns.

QUESTION: What are signs of depression in older people that EMTs should be aware of?
ANSWER: Depression might present as sadness, loss of interest in activities, unexplained weight loss or gain, insomnia or excessive sleep, feelings of worthlessness, or recurrent thoughts of death. These individuals may have a higher risk of suicide.

QUESTION: How does diabetes affect a geriatric patient's health and emergency care?
ANSWER: Diabetes can increase the risk of heart disease, kidney disease, vision loss, and poor wound healing. Hypoglycemia and hyperglycemia may present with altered mental status. Infections may be more severe.

QUESTION: What should EMTs be aware of when assessing and managing a patient with severe autism?
ANSWER: Patients with severe autism may be non-verbal, not respond to commands or questions, and hypersensitive to touch or sound. If possible, allow the patient to remain comfortable and involve caregivers in the assessment.

QUESTION: How should an EMT approach assessing and managing a patient with Alzheimer's disease?
ANSWER: The EMT should approach slowly and calmly, use simple language, repeat questions if necessary, involve caregivers in the assessment, and monitor the patient closely for changes in condition. These patients may be unable to provide a reliable history or understand instructions.

QUESTION: How does caring for a pediatric trauma patient differ from caring for an adult trauma patient?
ANSWER: In pediatric patients, there may be a delay in the presentation of shock, a lower capacity for blood loss, and a higher susceptibility to hypothermia. Assessment and interventions may need to be adapted to the child's size and developmental level.

EMS Operations

QUESTION: What is the primary purpose of an EMS system?
ANSWER: The primary purpose of an EMS system is to provide immediate medical care to those in need to prevent loss of life or aggravation of illness or injury.

QUESTION: Why is communication critical in EMS operations?
ANSWER: Communication is crucial in coordinating efforts among team members, relaying vital patient information to medical control, and ensuring a smooth transfer of care to the receiving facility.

QUESTION: What role does an EMT play in disaster response?
ANSWER: An EMT plays a critical role in disaster response by providing emergency medical care, triaging patients, evacuating casualties, and working in conjunction with other emergency services personnel.

QUESTION: How is patient triage performed in mass casualty incidents (MCI)?
ANSWER: In an MCI, patients are triaged based on the severity of their injuries, their likelihood of survival with immediate care, and available resources. The goal is to do the most good for the most people.

QUESTION: What is the role of the Incident Command System (ICS) in EMS operations?
ANSWER: The ICS provides a structured approach to incident management, allowing for a transparent chain of command, efficient resource allocation, and effective communication among all parties involved.

QUESTION: Why is it essential for EMS providers to use personal protective equipment (PPE)?
ANSWER: Using PPE protects EMS providers from exposure to infectious diseases, harmful chemicals, and physical dangers. It also helps prevent the spread of infection to other patients.

QUESTION: What steps should an EMT take if exposed to a patient's blood or bodily fluids?
ANSWER: If exposed, an EMT should immediately clean the area, notify their supervisor, complete an exposure report, and seek immediate medical attention for further evaluation and possible post-exposure prophylaxis.

QUESTION: How do protocols and standing orders contribute to EMS operations?
ANSWER: Protocols and standing orders guide an EMT's decision-making process and actions during a call. They are designed based on evidence-based practices to ensure optimal patient outcomes.

QUESTION: What considerations should be considered when lifting and moving a patient?
ANSWER: Safety is paramount. Providers should use proper lifting mechanics to avoid injury, consider the patient's condition and comfort, and choose the appropriate device for transport.

QUESTION: How does scene safety impact EMS operations?
ANSWER: Scene safety is essential to protect EMS providers from harm, enable effective patient care, and avoid exacerbating the patient's injuries or illness.

QUESTION: Why is thorough and accurate documentation essential in EMS operations?
ANSWER: Documentation provides a record of patient condition and care, helps with continuity of care, supports billing, provides data for quality improvement, and can serve as a legal record.

QUESTION: What are the special considerations when transferring care of a patient to hospital staff?
ANSWER: Accurate and concise information should be given to the receiving medical personnel, including patient identity, chief complaint, vital signs, treatment provided, and any changes during transport.

QUESTION: Why is continuing education and training important for EMTs?
ANSWER: Continuing education and training ensure that EMTs stay updated with the latest medical protocols, maintain their skills, and meet certification renewal requirements.

QUESTION: What is the role of EMS in public health?
ANSWER: EMS contributes to public health by providing emergency care, contributing to public health data, participating in prevention programs, and providing community education.

QUESTION: What are the responsibilities of an EMT at the scene of a motor vehicle collision?
ANSWER: Responsibilities include ensuring scene safety, assessing the patient, providing necessary care, coordinating with other emergency services, and arranging patient transport.

QUESTION: How does the "duty to act" concept apply to EMS professionals?
ANSWER: Duty to act refers to the obligation of EMS professionals to provide care if they are on duty, regardless of the circumstances. This includes responding to and appropriately managing emergencies.

QUESTION: How does an EMS system ensure quality assurance?
ANSWER: Quality assurance in EMS involves reviewing patient care reports for protocol adherence, analyzing outcomes, providing provider feedback, and adjusting protocols and training as necessary.

QUESTION: What considerations are considered when deciding to airlift a patient?
ANSWER: Considerations include the patient's condition, distance to the nearest appropriate hospital, traffic, and weather. Airlifting is typically reserved for critically ill or injured patients when time is crucial.

QUESTION: What is the role of dispatch in EMS operations?
ANSWER: Dispatch plays a critical role in receiving emergency calls, determining the nature and location of the emergency, dispatching the appropriate resources, and providing pre-arrival instructions to callers.

QUESTION: What are the key components of a thorough patient handoff at the hospital?
ANSWER: A thorough patient handoff includes an introduction, a summary of the patient's chief complaint and history of the present illness, vital signs and physical exam findings, treatment given, and the patient's response to treatment.

CONCLUSION

As we close this comprehensive guide designed to aid in your journey toward becoming an Emergency Medical Technician, we hope that it has equipped you with the foundational knowledge and understanding required to navigate the complexities of emergency medical services. Each chapter in this book, from Airway Management, through Patient Assessment, Medical Emergencies, Trauma, Special Populations, and finally, EMS Operations, was carefully crafted to provide a detailed view into the essential elements that make up the role of an EMT.

In Airway Management, you learned about the intricate anatomy and physiology of the respiratory system and mastered the techniques to maintain a clear and functioning airway, as well as oxygenation and ventilation.

The Patient Assessment chapter illuminated the systematic approach that every EMT must develop and fine-tune, which involves scene safety, initial assessment, detailed assessment, and ongoing assessment. This process is vital in determining a patient's condition, necessary treatment, and transport decisions.

When discussing Medical Emergencies, we delved into the pathophysiology, recognition, and management of various emergencies that an EMT may encounter, from cardiovascular to endocrine.

In the Trauma section, the focus shifted to injury assessment and management, including the different types of trauma and the specific techniques that are required to deal with them effectively.

The Special Populations chapter highlighted the unique considerations and adaptations necessary when treating specific demographic groups, including children, the elderly, and pregnant women.

Lastly, the EMS Operations chapter examined the operational aspects of being an EMT, from ambulance operations to disaster response, incident command systems, and handling mass casualty incidents.

Each section was developed to build a robust, well-rounded EMT who can adapt to various situations while providing exceptional patient care. Moreover, with the numerous questions and answers provided for each chapter, the objective was to create a critical-thinking EMT who knows the theory and can also apply it in practical scenarios.

As you move forward in your EMS journey, remember that this guide is only the beginning. The field of emergency medicine is dynamic, with new research, techniques, and equipment continually emerging. Lifelong learning, continuous skills practice, and a commitment to patient care are critical to your success as an EMT.

Finally, always remember the tremendous responsibility you carry as an EMT. You will often encounter people on their worst day, in their time of greatest need. Your knowledge, skills, and compassion can significantly impact their lives. Let this guide be the stepping stone to a fulfilling career in EMS, where every call is an opportunity to bring help, healing, and hope.

SPECIAL EXTRA CONTENT

Congratulations on Completing This Educational Journey!

Dear esteemed reader, If these final words are resonating with you, it signifies that you have successfully navigated through a path of personal and professional development, and we are privileged to have been part of your journey towards knowledge.

Your Insights Are Invaluable!

Your experiences, reflections, and feedback on the material you've just completed are crucial to us. We earnestly encourage you to share your thoughts about our book on Amazon. Whether a particular section struck a chord with you or the overall journey through the pages has broadened your understanding, your perspective is immensely important. By sharing your experiences, you help guide other learners and provide us, the authors, with the inspiration needed to refine our work and continue delivering impactful content.

Uncover Special EXTRA CONTENT Reserved Just for You!

In appreciation of your commitment, we've prepared exclusive additional content specifically for our readers. Here's what awaits you:

- **Audiobook** from listening to whenever and wherever you want!
- EBOOK of **Medical Terms**
- **Plunge into Real-World Crisis Management with Captivating Case Studies:** Supplement your theoretical knowledge with **25 riveting case studies**, each painting a vivid picture of real-world emergencies, ranging from multi-vehicle collisions to neonatal crises, from wilderness rescues to mass casualty incidents.
- **Comprehensive Guide to Common Drugs:** Our "Guide to Common Drugs" is an in-depth yet practical reference that walks you through over **50** commonly encountered medications in the field, from Aspirin to Zofran.
- **400 FLASHCARD!** You can track your progress and conveniently and interactively memorize the most important terms and concepts! Download to your device: **Anki APP or AnkiDroid**, or enter the web page and register free of charge. Then import the files we have given you as a gift and use the flashcards whenever and wherever you want to study and track your progress.

Straightforward Resources for Ongoing Enrichment

Below, you will find a distinctive QR CODE leading directly to your bonus content, ready for immediate download and exploration. There's no need for email subscriptions or personal detail disclosures; this is our direct gift to you, supporting your continued educational journey seamlessly.

Should you encounter any issues or have any questions regarding the downloadable material, please feel free to reach out to us at **booklovers.1001@gmail.com**
Sending warm regards and best wishes for your future endeavors.
With heartfelt thanks!

We look forward to your feedback!

Thank you!

Made in the USA
Las Vegas, NV
23 October 2024